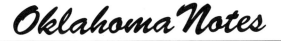

Oklahoma Notes

Clinical Sciences Review for Medical Licensure
Developed at
The University of Oklahoma College of Medicine

Ronald S. Krug, *Series Editor*

Suitable Reviews for:
United States Medical Licensing Examination
(USMLE), Step 2
Federation Licensing Examination (FLEX)

Oklahoma Notes

Internal Medicine

Dala R. Jarolim

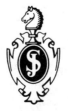

Springer-Verlag
New York Berlin Heidelberg London Paris
Tokyo Hong Kong Barcelona Budapest

Dala R. Jarolim, M.D. FACP
Department of Veteran Affairs
Medical Center
Muskogee, OK 74401
USA

Library of Congress Cataloging-in-Publication Data
Jarolim, Dala R.
    Oklahoma notes : internal medicine / Dala R. Jarolim.
      p.   cm. – (Oklahoma notes)
    ISBN 0-387-97960-3. – ISBN 3-540-97960-3
    1. Internal medicine–Examinations, questions, etc.   2. Internal
medicine–Outlines, syllabi, etc.   I. Title.   II. Title: Internal
medicine.   III. Series.
    [DNLM: 1. Internal Medicine–examination questions.   2. Internal
Medicine–outlines.   WB 18 J37o]
RC58.J37   1993
616'.0076–dc20
DNLM/DLC
for Library of Congress   92-48925
                                                                      CIP

Printed on acid-free paper.

Production managed by Jim Harbison; manufacturing supervised by Vincent Scelta.
Camera-ready copy prepared by the author.
Printed and bound by Edwards Brothers, Inc., Ann Arbor, MI.
Printed in the United States of America.

9 8 7 6 5 4 3

ISBN 0-387-97960-3 Springer-Verlag New York Berlin Heidelberg
ISBN 3-540-97960-3 Springer-Verlag Berlin Heidelberg New York

This book is dedicated to Oklahoma's legend, Richard A. Marshall, M.D., who taught me to love medicine, and to my husband, Reverend William L. Westmoreland, who taught me to love life.

Preface to the
Oklahoma Notes

In 1973 the University of Oklahoma College of Medicine instituted a requirement for passage of the Part 1 National Boards for promotion to the third year. To assist students in preparation for this examination a two-week review of the basic sciences was added to the Curriculum in 1975. Ten review texts were written by the faculty. In 1987 these basic science review texts were published as the *Oklahoma Notes* ("Okie Notes") and made available to all students of medicine who were preparing for comprehensive examinations. Over a quarter of a million of these texts have been sold nationally. Their clear, concise outline format has been found to be extremely useful by students preparing themselves for nationally standardized examinations.

Over the past few years numerous inquiries have been made regarding the availability of a Clinical Years series of "Okie Notes." Because of the obvious utility of the basic sciences books, faculty associated with the University of Oklahoma College of Medicine have developed texts in five specialty areas: Medicine, Neurology, Pediatrics, Psychiatry, and Surgery. Each of these texts follows the same condensed outline format as the basic science texts. The faculty who have prepared these texts are clinical educators and therefore the material incorporated in these texts has been validated in the classroom.

Each author has endeavored to distill the "need to know" material from their field of expertise. While preparing these texts, the target audience has always been the clinical years student who is preparing for Step 2 examinations.

A great deal of effort has gone into these texts. I hope they are helpful to you in studying for your licensure examinations.

Ronald S. Krug, Ph.D.
Series Editor

Preface

Congratulations on arriving at this stage in your medical career! This book is to help you condense the somewhat overwhelming constellation of Internal Medicine "facts" into a usable data base. It is not comprehensive and is obviously lopsided (for example, the Hematology and Oncology sections are expanded to take advantage of previously prepared material, and because students are often confused/intimidatd by the "C" word). It is not written by a basic scientist in the lab or a molecular biologist who rounds on the wards in May; rather the descriptors are of patients well-known from years in the trenches.

The covered subjects in this book are favorite topics of the "Professors of Medicine" around the country who write questions for standardized exams. Some topics in medicine come and go, some are cyclic, and some are classic. The latter should be your focus as you prepare for your next hurdle.

Many thanks to you, the student, for asking stimulating questions, for being so eager to learn, for working so hard, for making medicine fun for us, for carrying on the tradition!

Thanks to Karl Hoskison, M. D. for contributing questions.

Thanks to those who helped in the preparation of the manuscript: Barbara McCoy; Lorraine Marietta; my daugher, Debbie Baker; and Mariann Duca.

Enjoy, and may you never stop learning.

Dala R. Jarolim

Contents

CHAPTER 1: CARDIOLOGY

I. ARTERIAL HYPERTENSION

A. Surgically correctable causes
   Rare clinically but good for board exams

   1. Pheochromocytoma

      a. Volume depletion, intermittent hypertension, sweats, high glucose

      b. More common in men

      c. < 1% of all hypertensives. 10% bilateral, 10% extra adrenal, 10% malignant. May be familial.

      d. Do not tolerate anesthesia or surgery without treatment. Need to use alpha and beta blockers for norepinephrine and epinephrine excess.

   2. Aldosteronoma

      a. Low K+, autonomous production of aldosterone, suppressed renin.

      b. < 1% of all hypertensives.

   3. Renovascular

      a. Listen for bruit in belly

      b. Fibromuscular dysplasia amenable to angioplasty or surgery

        c. Atheromatous
common in patients with other evidence of atherosclerosis, diabetics.

   4. Coarctation of aorta

       a. In females with Turner's syndrome (XO); mainly males.

       b. Associated with other congenital cardiac lesions.

       c. CXR shows rib notching due to erosion from collateral intercostal vessels.

       d. "Machinery murmur" and asynchronous radial and femoral pulses on exam.

B. Essential

   1. Natural history (untreated)

       a. Patients are asymptomatic for years; see complications. Patients generally do not know when BP is high.

       b. Men: 20% survive 20 years.

       c. Women: 50% survive 20 years.

   2. Evidence for need to treat

       a. Treatment of hypertension decreases serious complications from 55% to 18%

       b. Decreased mortality when even mild hypertension is treated.

   3. Therapy

Increased BP and	Preferred Drug	Reason
CHF	ACE inhibitor	Unloads left ventricle acutely Decreases LV mass/volume chronically
Angina	Calcium channel blockers	Treats both

Increased BP and	Preferred Drug	Reason
Diabetes	ACE inhibitors	Reduces glomerular hypertension
Black	Thiazides	More effective than others
Elderly tendency to orthostasis	Clonidine	No orthostasis
Hyperlipidemia	Avoid beta blockers, thiazide	Exacerbate high lipids
Renal failure	Avoid thiazides	Does not work if creatinine > 2
Renal artery stenosis	Avoid ACE inhibitors	Worsens renal function
Myocardial infarct	Metoprolol	Decreased risk of second MI
Pregnancy	Alphamethyldopa	Old drug, safe
Mitral valve prolapse, anxiety, panic attacks, atrial fibrillation	Beta blockers	Calming effect, may decrease ectopics, control rate
Dissecting aortic aneurysm	Beta blockers; Apresoline is contraindicated unless above also used	Apresoline causes tachycardia, increases shear forces
Delirium tremens	Beta blockers, Clonidine	May help treat symptoms of DT's

C. Complications

  1. Cerebrovascular accident

     a. hemorrhagic - may have headache, loss of consciousness

     b. thrombotic - patient may awaken with hemiparesis. Commonly middle cerebral artery is occluded without loss of consciousness.

2. Atherosclerotic heart disease

3. Left ventricular hypertrophy, congestive heart failure

4. Chronic renal failure

5. Malignant hypertension (Hypertensive emergency). Cerebral edema and altered mental status, papilledema, proteinuria, micro-angiopathic anemia, pulmonary edema

6. Hypertensive urgency
   Proteinuria, renal failure, headache

7. Subarachnoid hemorrhage

   a. Sudden onset of severe headache ("the worst headache of my life"), stiff neck, loss of consciousness, focal neurologic deficits.

   b. CT positive for blood in 90%, need lumbar puncture to rule-in in other 10%.

8. Aortic aneurysm

   a. Diagnosis

      Feel belly for pulsatile mass, feel pulses. Listen for bruits. Consider surgery if > 6 cm wide due to high mortality if ruptured. Likelihood of rupture increases if > 6 cm.

   b. Aortic dissection

      Patient complains of pain radiating to back. Pulses may be absent, limbs may be cool or cyanotic, decreased urine output, hypo-tension, tachycardia. Look for widening of mediastinum on chest x-ray, calcium in walls of aorta on abdominal film, size of aneurysm on KUB, ultrasound or CT scan.

II. CORONARY ARTERY DISEASE

A. Epidemiology

1. Steady decline in death rate since 1965 (45% decrease). Still one-third of deaths or 600,000 annually.

2. Risk factors: hypercholesterolemia, hypertension, cigarette smoking, diabetes, family history, physical inactivity, obesity, menopause for women, male sex.

B. Angina Pectoris

1. Symptoms and signs

   a. Classically dull substernal chest pain, pressure or heaviness, tightness with radiation to left shoulder, neck and associated dyspnea, nausea, diaphoresis.

   b. Occurs with exercise, relieved with rest.

   c. Levine's sign (Clenched fist over sternum).

   d. S4, increased BP, EKG may show ST depression, change in heart rate.

2. Treatment

   a. Medical

      1. Nitrates

         Sublingual tablets, spray
         Oral
         Patch
         IV for unstable angina

      2. Calcium channel blockers

      3. Beta blockers

      4. Aspirin

      5. Heparin for unstable angina

      6. Reduce risk factors: stop smoking, decrease cholesterol, control BP, weight loss, graded exercise

   b. Surgical: angioplasty, coronary artery bypass

C. Myocardial Infarction

1. Diagnosis: high index of suspicion, history important! Must exclude even if (-) EKG.

2. Treatment: thrombolysis, treat arrhythmias, ASA, heparin, angioplasty, beta blockers

3. Cardiogenic shock: dobutamine, fluids if dry, balloon pump

4. Secondary prevention

   a. modification of risk factors

   b. cholesterol: lowering by 1% decreases risk of MI by 2%

D. Chest Pain Syndromes

Unstable angina   Costochondritis
Stable angina   Intercostal muscle spasm
Prinzmetal's angina   Cervical disk disease
Esophageal spasm   Pleurisy
Esophageal reflux   Pulmonary hypertension
Pneumonia   Pulmonary embolus
Myocardial infarction   Lung cancer
Pericarditis

E. Clinical Pearl

angor animi - sense of impending doom in MI, PE. Listen to your patient if he says he's going to die!

III. **CONGENITAL HEART DISEASE**

A. Know

1. Pulmonary hypertension - vasoactive pulmonary bed, the response of which determines the clinical findings and prognosis in congenital heart disease.

2. Right to left shunts - associated with arterial oxygen desaturation and cyanosis, the degree being related to magnitude of pulmonary blood flow. The latter may be decreased (Tetralogy) or increased (transposition of great vessels).

3. Eisenmenger's syndrome or physiology - a term applied to a condition which occurs in several congenital diseases where pulmonary hypertension develops; a previous left to right shunt reverses to right to left. The systemic blood then is desaturated with non-oxygenated blood,

cyanosis and clubbing develop, and dyspnea and fatigue worsen. The goal of surgical treatment is to intervene before the syndrome occurs because when well established, it is irreversible and fatal.

B. Major Congenital Lesions

1. Atrial septal defect

   a. Females > males. Dyspnea on exertion. L parasternal lift, L sternal systolic ejection murmur, widely split fixed S2.

   b. EKG shows R axis deviation and R ventricular hypertrophy. (If L axis, think primum)

   c. CXR shows enlarged R atrium, R ventricle and pulmonary artery

   d. Cardiac catheterization localizes shunt by step-up in oxygen concentration between vena cava and R atrium

   e. ASD needs to be surgically corrected even in adults unless shunt has reversed to R to L (then it is too late).

   f. Atrial arrhythmias common

   g. Types of ASD

      1. primum ASD - (endocardial cushion defect). Associated mitral regurgitation; left axis deviation on EKG, right ventricular and occasional L ventricular hypertrophy. Cardiac catheterization shows "goose-neck" deformity of abnormally placed mitral valve.

      2. secundum ASD - common congenital lesion in adults, L to R shunt. Echocardiogram shows enlarged end diastolic dimension of R ventricle, enlarged R atrium. Doppler shows flow disturbance.

2. Ventricular septal defect (VSD)

   a. most common form of congenital heart disease

   b. perimembranous defect most frequent VSD

    c. small defects

        1. usually close spontaneously

        2. palpable systolic thrill, harsh pansystolic murmur

        3. usually normal EKG, CXR, echocardiogram (Doppler can pick up shunt)

    d. large defects

        1. rare in adults

        2. large left to right shunts, then increased pulmonary vascular resistance, left ventricular failure, shunt reversal, right ventricular failure

        3. if associated pulmonic stenosis limits pulmonic blood flow, babies may improve

        4. surgery usually indicated

3. Tetralogy of Fallot

    a. four defects

        1. R ventricular outflow tract obstruction (pulmonic stenosis)

        2. VSD

        3. overriding of aorta above VSD

        4. right ventricular hypertrophy

    b. Severe R ventricular outflow tract obstruction decreases pulmonary blood flow and unoxygenated blood is shunted across VSD to systemic circulation. Cyanosis and dyspnea on exertion result.

    c. Squatting is seen in children at play and reduces R to L shunt by increasing systemic vascular resistance and pulmonary blood flow.

    d. Normal heart size, tapping apical impulse due to enlarged R ventricle, widely radiating systolic murmur which decreases with severe obstruction, aortic ejection click, single S2, clubbing, cyanosis, growth retardation.

e. CXR shows normal heart size, elevation of cardiac apex, large aorta, decreased pulmonary vasculature.

f. EKG shows R axis deviation and R ventricular hypertrophy.

g. Echocardiogram shows the tetralogy.

h. Cardiac catheterization shows identical systolic pressures in both ventricles, significant gradient ventricular outflow, decreased arterial oxygen saturation.

i. Surgically treated during childhood.

j. Common in Down's syndrome.

4. Ebstein's Anomaly

a. Tricuspid valve is displaced into R ventricle.

b. "Atrialized R ventricle" refers to thin portion of ventricle proximal to tricuspid valve.

c. Tricuspid regurgitation causes increased R atrial pressure and R to L shunt across atrial septum (ASD or patent foramen) with cyanosis.

d. Paroxysmal atrial tachycardia, multiple murmurs, clicks, S3, S4, opening snap of tricuspid valve.

e. EKG shows R bundle branch block, large P waves, prolonged P-R interval.

5. Patent ductus arteriosus

a. Females > males, prematurity, maternal rubella

b. Usually asymptomatic, usually small flow through ductus, thus normal pulmonary arterial pressure

c. continuous murmur

d. if shunt reversed, cyanosis of lower extremities occurs

e. EKG shows L ventricular hypertrophy if large flow, R ventricular hypertrophy if severe pulmonary hypertension

f. confirm with echocardiogram

g. surgical correction advised

6. Bicuspid aortic valve

a. occurs in 2% of population

b. 2 commissures, 2 cusps

c. may function normally for life, or

d. may develop fibrotic thickened calcified leaflets and cause aortic stenosis

e. may develop prolapse or eversion with aortic regurgitation (diastolic murmur)

f. marked predisposition to bacterial endocarditis

g. listen for short soft systolic murmur and early aortic ejection click

7. Asymmetric septal hypertrophy

a. genetic transmission

b. cellular disarray histologically

c. syncope or sudden death in previously healthy young persons during strenuous exertion

d. dyspnea, fatigue, angina-type pain

e. prominent apical impulse and A waves, S4, occasional paradoxically split S2, systolic murmur loudest at apex with radiation to axilla, seldom to neck. If LV cavity size decreases, gradient increases and vice versa.

Increased gradient (increased murmur)	Decreased gradient (decreased murmur)
Valsalva straining Rising from squatting Compensatory pause After premature beat Isotonic exercise, Amylnitrate, nitro- glycerin, digitalis	Valsalva release Squatting Isometric exercise (handgrip, beta- blockade)

Hence the use of beta blockers to treat and the avoidance of digitalis.

IV. VALVULAR HEART DISEASE

Onset of murmurs:

In childhood, think congenital;
In young adults, think rheumatic or hypertrophic;
In elderly, think degenerative

A. Aortic Stenosis

1. Symptoms

    a. Early - none; diagnosis suspected by scratchy, harsh systolic murmur at apex to sternal notch to carotids.

    b. Late - angina, syncope, secondary to complete heart block, CHF. 2 year 50% mortality without surgery. Men > women.

2. Physical findings

    a. murmur as above

    b. slow carotid upstroke

    c. left ventricular hypertrophy with apical impulse displaced to left

3. EKG

    Left ventricular hypertrophy.

4. Treatment

   Valve replacement when symptomatic or valve orifice < .5 cm2.

B. Aortic Insufficiency

   1. Volume overload of L ventricle.

   2. Develops gradually, well tolerated for years.

   3. Etiologies:

      Rheumatic fever
      Degenerative
        bicuspid valve
        myxomatous
        cystic medial necrosis
      Aneurysms of sinus of
        Valsalva
      Infectious
        endocarditis with
        perforated cusp,
        syphilis

      Rheumatic diseases
        Reiter's syndrome,
        ankylosing spon-
        dylitis
        rheumatoid arthri-
        tis
      Hereditable
        Marfan's
      Prosthetic valve
      Hypertension

   4. Symptoms relate to development of congestive heart failure

   5. Signs are of hyperdynamic circulation: active precordium, bounding pulses, head bobbing with pulse; high pitched blowing decrescendo diastolic murmur heard best over left sternal border with patient sitting up, leaning forward, in expiration

   6. Surgical treatment is indicated before the left ventricle is irreversibly dilated. Follow the size of LV by echocardiogram.

      One previously used criterion for surgery is an end-systolic LV dimension of 55 mm

   7. Acute aortic regurgitation

      a. sudden LV pressure and volume overload result in pulmonary edema in face of normal heart size

      b. urgent surgery required. Use preload and afterload reducers while arranging surgery.

C. Mitral Stenosis

    1. Symptoms

       dyspnea, cough, women > men, hemoptysis, history of rheumatic fever

    2. Physical findings

       Pulmonary congestion: rales, engorged neck veins; hemoptysis; often atrial fibrillation; diastolic rumbling murmur in left lateral decubitus position. Evidence of embolic phenomena.

    3. EKG shows left atrial hypertrophy, right ventricular hypertrophy. Echocardiogram shows square wave motion of E to F slope during diastole.

    4. Surgical treatment

       a. mitral valve commissurotomy if valve pliable

       b. mitral valve replacement - many patients are women of child bearing age. A prosthetic valve commits them to lifelong Coumadin, which is teratogenic. A porcine valve does not, though it has a finite life span and will need replacement.

       c. Timing based on development of symptoms

D. Mitral Insufficiency

    1. Symptoms

       a. may be well tolerated due to chronic slow LV volume overload, dilatation and hypertrophy. Fatigue and dyspnea develop as LV decompensates.

       b. If acute, pressure overload of LV leads to acute pulmonary edema. Urgent surgery may be required. Reduce preload and afterload while arranging for surgery.

    2. Physical findings: cardiomegaly with enlarged LV; holosystolic murmur radiating to axilla, S3, soft S1.

3. Chronic mitral <u>regurgitation</u>	Acute mitral <u>regurgitation</u>
Rheumatic	Ruptured chordae tendinae
Myxomatous	(MI or endocarditis)
Mitral valve prolapse	Ruptured papillary muscle (same)
Degenerative annular calcification	Perforation of leaflet Prosthetic valve
Connective tissue	
Coronary disease	
Prosthetic valve	

E. Mitral valve prolapse

1. Usually not a serious clinical problem. Women > men, young, anxious. "Click-murmur syndrome."

2. May have chest pain, palpitations, fatigue.

3. Echocardiogram shows prolapse in 5% adults. May not agree with physical exam.

4. Prophylax for endocarditis if click and murmur. Look for other psychophysiologic problems, reassure. If symptomatic ventricular ectopy, beta blockers.

V. **ENDOCARDITIS**

A. Symptoms

1. Of multi-system disease: can have CVA's, arthralgia, renal failure; do have fever.

2. Can be confused with connective tissue disease or other infectious disease.

B. Physical findings:

1. Signs of emboli such as Roth spots in fundi, Janeway lesions on palms and soles, Osler's nodes in pads of fingers, petechiae; changing murmurs.

2. Source of emboli: heart valve vegetations, endocardial vegetations common in congenital heart disease.

C. Etiologies of Endocarditis

1. Rheumatic - Streptococcus viridans after dental work

2. Staphylococcus aureus (especially coagulase negative) after prosthetic devices such as IV lines

3. Enterococcus after GU instrumentation.

4. IV drug users - Often get right sided endocarditis with septic pulmonary emboli due to staphylococcus aureus, coagulase positive.

5. Prosthetic valve - staph coagulase positive and negative, fungal

6. Congenital heart disease - similar to rheumatic

7. Culture negative 5-10%

8. Marantic - (non-bacterial thrombotic endocarditis), seen with mucin producing adenocarcinomas

D. Treatment: identify organism, treat medically. May need surgery to cure.

VI. **PERICARDITIS**

A. Symptoms

1. Chest pain, dyspnea.

2. Pain is better when sitting up, leaning forward

B. Physical Findings

1. Three component pericardial friction rub, may have fever.

2. May have coexisting pleural effusion.

C. Studies

1. EKG shows diffuse ST segment elevation.

2. Echocardiogram shows pericardial effusion (echo-free space).

3. CXR to help exclude lung cancer.

4. PPD to help exclude tuberculosis.

5. Pericardial fluid may be obtained for culture, cytology.

6. ANA if drug induced lupus or systemic lupus a possibility.

D. Etiologies

1. Viral

2. Bacterial: with infected devices.

3. Post myocardial infarction

4. Post cardiotomy: Dressler's Syndrome

5. Connective tissue diseases: lupus, rheumatoid arthritis, scleroderma

6. Drug induced: procainamide, hydralazine

7. Malignant: lung cancer

E. Treatment

Nonsteroidals, steroids if severe, pericardial window if tamponade.

VII. TAMPONADE

A. Symptoms

chest tightness, dyspnea

B. Signs

Increased neck veins, hypotension, pulsus paradoxicus, enlarged heart on CXR

C. EKG shows electrical alternans of P wave, QRS complex, and T wave.

D. Confirm with echocardiogram showing R atrial compression, diastolic collapse of R ventricle, pendular swinging of heart in pericardial fluid. Treat with fluids, pericardiocentesis, window

VIII. ANTICOAGULATION

A. Contraindications to anticoagulation: recent CVA (hemorrhagic or thrombotic), GI bleeding, pericarditis, malignant hypertension, severe thrombocytopenia, proliferative diabetic retinopathy, post partum.

B. Candidates for anticoagulation 1992: acute myocardial infarction (after thrombolysis or if not done), unstable angina, embolic stroke, left ventricular or atrial thrombus, chronic atrial fibrillation, deep venous thrombosis, pulmonary embolism, transient ischemic attack refractory to aspirin and Ticlid.

IX. CONGESTIVE HEART FAILURE

A. Symptoms

Breathlessness, lower extremity swelling, fatigue, dyspnea on exertion, paroxysmal nocturnal dyspnea

B. Physical Findings

Cardiomegaly (laterally displaced apical impulse), tachycardia, S3 gallop, wheezes (cardiac asthma), hepatomegaly, pretibial and pedal edema, engorged neck veins, conversational dyspnea.

C. Etiologies

1. Ischemic cardiomyopathy

2. Hypertrophic cardiomyopathy

3. Restrictive cardiomyopathy

a. Infiltrative

amyloid, sarcoid, hemochromatosis, metabolic, inherited diseases

      b.   Non-infiltrative

           radiation (delayed maybe up to 10 years), connective tissue diseases

4.   Alcoholic cardiomyopathy

5.   Valvular heart disease

6.   Myocardial infarction

7.   Nutritional (beri beri)

8.   Cor pulmonale

9.   Arrhythmias

D. Treatment

Diuretics, ACE inhibitors, nitroprusside, salt and water restriction, dobutamine, other inotropes, digitalis, balloon pump, correction of any surgical cause; intubation with mechanical ventilation. Management of very sick patient facilitated by Swan Ganz monitoring of left atrial and pulmonary artery pressures.

X. **ARRHYTHMIAS**

A. Atrial

1.   Premature atrial contractions may occur with digitalis toxicity, may precipitate paroxysmal atrial tachycardia, or atrial flutter; not usually a clinical problem.

2.   Paroxysmal atrial tachycardia has sudden start and end. Seen in alcoholics after binge drinking ("holiday heart"), and in hyperthyroidism.

3.   Atrial fibrillation with irregularly irregular rhythm. Common in pulmonary embolus, hyperthyroidism, mitral valve disease. If very slow (50's), think of digitalis toxicity.

4.   Atrial flutter may occur alone or with intermittent atrial fibrillation (fib-flutter). Get echo to rule out mitral valve disease.

5.   Multifocal atrial tachycardia most common arrhythmia in COPD.

B. Ventricular

1. Premature ventricular contractions - worrisome characteristics: > 6/min, multiform, "R on T' phenomenon after acute MI could lead to ventricular tachycardia or fibrillation. Are a marker long term after MI for continuing ischemia, but suppression with some recently tested agents leads to increased mortality.

2. Ventricular tachycardia:

   Asymptomatic: no syncope or dizziness, no blood pressure changes. Usually of short duration.

   Symptomatic: with above, or if sustained, needs suppression. Common in cardiomyopathies.

3. "Sick sinus syndrome" - alternating tachy-arrhythmias and bradycardia, often with long pauses, complete heart block. Treated with drugs for former and pacemaker for latter.

4. Complete heart block:

   a. slow rate, chronic: patient may have time to compensate and present in chronic congestive heart failure.

   b. acutely after MI: requires pacer, worse prognosis, anticipate in patients with lesser blocks as left anterior hemiblock, left bundle branch block, first degree A-V block.

   c. Congenital syndromes:

      1. in infants of mothers with lupus.

      2. familial with usually good prognosis; pace if syncope occurs.

   d. Iatrogenic from beta blockers, calcium blockers.

5. Torsades de pointe:

   a. common with quinidine and procainamide

   b. patients with prolonged Q-T interval are at risk

    c. recognize the syndrome, remove drug, treat with isoproterenol or overdrive pacing to terminate.

6. Digitalis toxic rhythms

    a. Atrial tachycardia with block.

    b. Non-paroxysmal AV junctional tachycardia.

    c. AV block.

    d. Ventricular tachycardia.

    e. Treat by eliminating drug, using potassium, Lidocaine, phenytoin or pacemaker as needed.

XI.   QUESTIONS

Patient 1:   (Questions 1 through 4)

A 23-year-old female is brought to the emergency room after complaining of a severe headache (the worst in her life) and collapsing. Exam reveals stupor, BP 230/110, T 97, P 100, R 26, meningismus, subhyaloid hemorrhage on fundoscopic, systolic murmur over anterior chest becoming continuous over the back, delayed femoral pulsations and wide carrying angle of the arms (You notice this and confirm with family).

1. The single best explanation for her acute event is:

    a. migraine headache
    b. thrombotic CVA
    c. endocarditis
    d. subarachnoid hemorrhage
    e. hypertensive encephalopathy

2. The best explanation of her murmurs is:

    a. aortic stenosis and insufficiency
    b. mitral stenosis and insufficiency
    c. atrial septal defect
    d. ventricular septal defect
    e. coarctation of the aorta

3. The best explanation anatomically for her acute event is:

   a. aneurysm of the circle of Willis with bleeding into subarachnoid space
   b. vegetation on the aortic valve
   c. clot in the middle cerebral artery
   d. vasoconstriction
   e. neuronal spreading depression.

4. Her congenital condition which ties the clinical picture together is:

   a. Down's syndrome
   b. Apert's syndrome
   c. Turner's syndrome
   d. Polyglandular endocrinopathy
   e. Neurofibromatosis

Patient 2: (Questions 5 and 6)

A 79-year-old white male presents with witnessed syncope (no seizure activity) and dyspnea. Exam reveals BP 180/100, P 60's with pauses, T 98 R 20; systolic scratchy harsh murmur over precordium radiating to sternal notch and carotids; displaced apical impulse, rales bilaterally. Monitor shows occasional 2 second pauses; EKG shows LVH and complete heart block.

5. The next best test to work up this patient's problem is:

   a. EEG
   b. Echocardiogram
   c. CT brain scan
   d. Right heart catheter
   e. Pulmonary functions

6. You find something surgically correctable on this test. In discussing the need for surgery with this patient you need to understand

   a. Surgery is for cosmetic reasons only.
   b. Surgery will improve quality of life, not quantity.
   c. Surgery is indicated only for young patients.
   d. Surgery is associated with a 50% mortality.
   e. Untreated surgically, the pt has a 50% two year survival.

Patient 3: (Question 7)

A 50-year-old male patient complains in April of choking sensations at night which awaken him and force him to sit upright while sleeping. He has smoked for 40 years and his 67 year old mother died recently of a CVA secondary to hypertension. Exam reveals BP 190/90, P 100, weight 278. few basilar rales, laterally displaced PMI, frequent ectopic beats, 2+ pitting edema. EKG reveals LVH and bilateral enlargement. CXR shows mild cardiac enlargement, fluid in fissures. While discussing these abnormal findings, you witness one of these episodes while the pt is sitting down.

7. The best explanation for the patient's symptoms is:

   a. Allergic rhinitis
   b. Exacerbation of COPD
   c. Sleep apnea syndrome
   d. Intermittent LV dysfunction
   e. Reflux esophagitis

Patient 4: (Questions 8 and 9)

A 25-year-old Hispanic male from a large Eastern city is admitted with fever and malaise. On exam you note a temperature of 103 degrees, palatal and conjunctival petechiae, a systolic grade III/VI murmur along LSB, tenderness and fullness of LUQ and track marks with cellulitis over antecubital fossae and forearms of hands.

8. You order the appropriate tests which include all but:

   a. blood cultures
   b. chest Xray
   c. CBC
   d. liver biopsy
   e. echocardiogram

9. After he arrives on the floor his blood pressure which had been 120/80 changes to 140/50, his heart rate increases from 100 to 120 and he becomes pale and diaphoretic as he complains of chest pain. Auscultation of his heart reveals a new soft, short diastolic murmur more prominent as he leans forward. What has happened?

    a. Myocardial infarction
    b. Pericarditis
    c. Septic embolus to spleen
    d. Perforated aortic cusps
    e. Exacerbation of rheumatic heart disease

Patient 5: (Questions 10 through 12)

A 45-year-old white female underwent cholecystectomy and on day two became acutely dyspneic after straining to pass gas. She became tachypneic, tachycardic and diaphoretic. She had a few expiratory wheezes bilaterally. A blood gas revealed pH 7.50 pCO2 25 pO2 60. CXR was unremarkable.

10. The most likely explanation for her acute problem is:

    a. myocardial infarction
    b. pulmonary embolus
    c. post operative ileus
    d. sepsis from wound infection
    e. gallstone ileus

11. You manage the pt medically and she stabilizes. After several days she develops gangrenous areas over the lateral thighs. The most likely cause of this new problem is:

    a. Embolization to and infarction of skin from infective endocarditis.
    b. Development of necrotizing fasciitis from a gangrenous gallbladder.
    c. Pressure necrosis from bed rest
    d. Allergic reaction to a cephalosporin
    e. Coumadin skin necrosis

12. An underlying abnormal protein is searched for. You
    want to know her levels of:

    a. Protein S
    b. Protein C
    c. Rheumatoid factor
    d. ANA
    e. Antithrombin III

13. The most common cause of sudden death is

    a. arrhythmias
    b. ruptured myocardium
    c. electromechanical dissociation
    d. massive pulmonary embolus

14. Placement of the Swan-Ganz catheter has the following
    potential complications

    a. ventricular ectopy
    b. right bundle branch block pattern
    c. perforation of the pulmonary artery
    d. pulmonary infarction
    e. all of the above

15. The most common side-effect of nitroglycerin prepara-
    tions is

    a. diarrhea
    b. pounding headache
    c. nausea
    d. chest pain

16. The patient had an irregularly irregular heart rate
    of 140 beats per minute, but his vital signs were
    stable. The most probable dysrhythmia in this
    patient would be

    a. ventricular tachycardia
    b. ventricular fibrillation
    c. atrial fibrillation
    d. sinus tachycardia

17. Which of the following valvular heart lesions produces a loud, snapping S1, an opening snap, and a diastolic rumble?

    a. mitral stenosis
    b. mitral regurgitation
    c. aortic stenosis
    d. aortic regurgitation

18. Coxsackie B virus is the most common cause of acute myocarditis in the United States, associated with fever, arrhythmias, chest pain, and possibly transient congestive heart failure.

    _____ True   _____ False

19. A common acute stress on the myocardium that precipitates congestive heart failure is

    a. acute volume or salt load
    b. ischemia or infarction
    c. uncontrolled hypertension
    d. hyperthyroidism
    e. all of the above

20. Uncommon causes of hypertension include

    a. pheochromocytoma
    b. Conn's syndrome of aldosterone secreting adrenal adenoma
    c. renal artery stenosis
    d. coarctation of the aorta
    e. all of the above

21. The drug of choice in a life-threatening hypertensive crisis is

    a. nitroprusside intravenously
    b. beta blockers
    c. nifedipine
    d. ACE inhibitors

22. The most common cause of stroke in this country is

    a. hemorrhage
    b. arterial thrombosis
    c. cardiac source emboli
    d. trauma

23. Lacunar strokes are a family of syndromes that occur in patients with hypertension and atherosclerosis.

    _____ True   _____ False

24. The most probable etiology of acute stroke in a patient with atrial fibrillation, mitral stenosis, dilated cardiomyopathy or ventricular aneurysm would be

    a. thrombotic
    b. embolic
    c. hemorrhagic

25. A transient ischemic attack (TIA) presents as an acute neurological deficit that must resolve (by definition) within

    a. one month
    b. seven days
    c. three days
    d. 24 hours

26. Approximately 25 percent of patients with TIA's suffer a cerebrovascular accident within five days and often within the first month of the first transient ischemic attack.

    _____ True   _____ False

XII. ANSWERS

1. d   This is the presentation of acute subarachnoid hemorrhage. Varying levels of coma may be present with prognosis declining as grade increases.

2. e   The exam of the cardiovascular system reveals findings of coarctation. The murmur posteriorly is from increased blood flow through intercostal vessels. The latter leads to rib notching on CXR.

3. a   Most subarachnoid hemorrhages occur from aneurysms in this location. Turner's syndrome patients have associated multiple cerebral aneurysms and coarctation of the aorta.

4. c

5. b   An echocardiogram quickly confirms the clinical diagnosis of aortic stenosis and gives an estimate of the severity. With a valve orifice area of $< .5$ cm^2 and the clinical symptoms of syncope secondary to heart block (Stokes-Adams), valve replacement is indicated.

6. e   When symptoms of angina, syncope or CHF develop in a patient with aortic stenosis, the life expectancy is 50% at two years.

7. d   Cough and upper respiratory congestion in the spring can often be due to allergic rhinitis and asthma. However, the risk factors for and physical findings of heart disease demand that it be considered. The pt had on his own sought an allergy consultation and had negative skin tests.

The patient's nocturnal symptoms and obesity speak for sleep apnea. However, they also were witnessed in the day-time while sitting (not recumbent). Most sleep apnea patients complain of daytime somnolence not nighttime events. The pt could have COPD with his long smoking history. The cough was non productive; the Xray did not show increased A-P diameter or flattened diaphragms.

The patient's girth and recumbent symptoms could suggest gastroesophageal reflux disease (GERD). Cough can be prominent in this symptom complex. However, LV dysfunction in this pt caused his paroxysmal nocturnal dyspnea and his angina-equivalent during the stressful conversation regarding his health. He improved with diuretics and calcium channel blockers.

8. d   This injection drug user has acute endocarditis as manifested by signs of embolization, fever, and murmur. All answers are appropriate for initial work-up of this condition except liver biopsy. He may well have liver disease as a sequel to hepatitis B or C from IV drug use, but the liver would not be biopsied on day one.

9. e   The dreaded complication of perforated aortic cusps occurred with the pt developing acute aortic insufficiency. Urgent management includes consideration of valve replacement.

10. b   Pulmonary emboli are very common after chole-stectomy. Pre-op low dose subcutaneous heparin can decrease the incidence.

11. e   Coumadin skin necrosis occurs in predisposed individuals in areas of adipose tissue. It occurs in protein C deficient patients when Coumadin is given before adequate heparin therapy has raised levels of anti-thrombin III.

12. b

13. a

14. e

15. b

16. c

17. a

18. True

19. e

20. e

21. a

22. b

23. True

24. b

25. d

26. True

CHAPTER 2: RESPIRATORY DISEASES

I. CHRONIC OBSTRUCTIVE PULMONARY DISEASE

A. Symptoms

Dyspnea on exertion, cough, sputum production, breath-lessness

B. Physical Findings

Apical impulse in epigastrium, fixed barrel chest, increased AP diameter, distant heart tones, tachy-cardia, wheezes, rales. May have cyanosis, pedal edema, engorged neck veins.

C. Chronic Bronchitis

1. Definition: 1/2 cup sputum daily for three months out of the year for two years.

2. Usually smoking related

3. Clinical features of "blue bloaters"

   a. Cough, sputum, wheezing, frequent respiratory infections

   b. Recurrent attacks of acute bronchitis which bring patient to medical attention; patient gets hypoxemic with these

   c. Commonly obese, edematous

   d. Retain CO_2, get cyanotic especially with acute episodes

   e. Respond to bronchodilators, steroids, oxygen

      f.   Commonly associated with sleep apnea syndromes

      g.   Many opportunities for you to give the stop smoking message

      h.   Constant decline in pulmonary functions (FEV1) over years (40-45 ml/year compared to 20-25 ml/year in non-smoker)

D.   Emphysema

   1.   <u>Panacinar</u> due to <u>alpha-1-antitrypsin deficiency</u> (more often lower lobes)

      a.   "Pi" (protein inhibitor) phenotype determines susceptibility, normals are homozygous for allele MM at Pi locus (PiMM).

      b.   If patient is Pi ZZ, alpha 1 antitrypsin levels are reduced and disease develops.

      c.   Heterozygotes Pi MZ do not get emphysema despite some reduction in enzyme levels. They are at higher risk for liver disease than MM.

      d.   Alpha 1 antitrypsin deficiency is autosomal recessive.

      e.   Emphysema develops by age 60 in nonsmoking homozygotes and by age 40 in smoking homozygotes, who sustain a 150 ml decline in FEV1 yearly.

   2.   <u>Centrilobular</u> due to smoking (more upper lobes)

      a.   Progressive loss of alveoli thought to be due to proteolytic enzymes and their stimulation by cigarette smoke

      b.   Clinical features of "pink puffer"

         1.   Little wheezing or sputum

         2.   Maintains a fairly decent pO2 until late in course due to hyperventilation

         3.   Usually thin body habitus, minimal edema until late

   4.   Breathlessness   is the primary symptom,
        occurs late.   Usually non responsive to
        bronchodilators.

   5.   Cor   pulmonale,   secondary   polycythemia
        develop.

   6.   Correlation of FEV1 with survival:

        FEV1 > 1.2 liters, 10 year survival
        FEV1 = 1.0 liters, 5 year survival
        FEV1 < 700 cc, 2 year survival

E.   Smoking

   Tell your patients they must stop (this works).

F.   Treatment

   Oxygen, inhaled steroids, inhaled and oral beta 2
   agonists, theophylline, treat infections, treat
   coexisting heart disease, pulmonary toilet, exercise.

G.   Causes of Increased Dyspnea in COPD

   When a stable COPD patient gets worse, think of these
   things

   Pneumothorax   Pneumonia
   Pneumomediastinum   Bronchitis
   Pulmonary embolus   Heart failure, left sided
   Mucus plugging   Allergic component
   Anemia   Restrictive component
   Arrhythmia   Electrolyte abnormality
   Cor pulmonale   Myocardial ischemia or
   Tuberculosis   infarction

H.   Caution

   Do not exceed 1-2 liters/min O2 in CO2 retainers.
   They depend on their hypoxemia to stimulate
   respiration, and raising the pO2 may cause respiratory depression, further CO2 retention, and
   death.

   Pearls:

   1.   O2 is the best diuretic

   2.   Multifocal atrial tachycardia is the most common
        arrhythmia in COPD.

3. GI bleeding due to stress is very frequent in lung patient on ventilator

4. Causes of failure to wean from ventilator:

   a. metabolic alkalosis occurs often in intubated patient on diuretics

   b. muscles weaken due to catabolism and lack of nutrition

   c. coexisting heart failure, pulmonary embolism, hypothyroidism (see list in G)

II. ASTHMA

A. Symptoms

Reversible chest tightness, cough, wheeze, dyspnea in paroxysms. May be triggered by allergens, exercise, cold, viruses, laughing, emotions.

B. Physical Findings During Attack

Wheezes, increased neck veins, use of accessory muscles of respiration, air trapping with flattened diaphragms, cyanosis, anxiety, tachycardia, tachypnea.

C. Etiologies

1. Intrinsic: onset young to middle adult life; may have nasal polyps and aspirin sensitivity. Know this.

2. Extrinsic: react to allergens (pollens, mold, house mites), cold, exercise, smoke

3. Occupational, especially toluene isocyanate

D. Treatment

1. Inhaled steroids

2. Inhaled bronchodilators

3. Oral bronchodilators

4. Oral, IV steroids

5. Avoidance of precipitating triggers.

E. Death in young asthmatics is on the rise over the last decade.   Undertreating and overtreating with beta stimulants have both been blamed.   An asthmatic is hypocapneic early in an attack, but with fatigue may start to retain pCO2.   This is an ominous sign and requires intensive therapy.

III. SLEEP APNEA SYNDROMES

A. Central - rare

B. Obstructive Symptoms

  1. Excessive daytime somnolence, forgetfulness, decreased concentration; excessive nocturnal snoring, "so bad that wife sleeps in other room."

  2. Signs: obesity, pedal edema, excess oropharyngeal tissue.

C. Diagnose with sleep study looking for airway obstructive events with hypoxemia.

D. Treatment

  1. Assess for efficacy of nocturnal nasal C-PAP

  2. Weight loss

  3. Pharyngoplasty, tracheostomy

IV. PULMONARY EMBOLISM

A. Symptoms

Breathlessness, anxiety, air hunger, chest pain

B. Physical Findings

Tachycardia, tachypnea, localized wheeze; can have hypotension, diaphoresis, may have splinting with infarction

C. Risk Factors - know this:

Postoperative, especially orthopedic
Obesity
Stasis
Pregnancy, oral contraceptives
Congestive heart failure
Lupus "anticoagulant" and anticardiolipin antibodies
Malignancy
Hypercoagulable familial states

1. Protein C deficiency. In homozygous protein C deficiency when Coumadin is begun, the concentration of protein C, a natural anticoagulant, falls more rapidly than clotting factors II, IX and X, inducing a hypercoagulable state. Necrosis occurs in skin over adipose tissue such as breasts and thighs.

2. Protein S Deficiency.

3. Antithrombin III Deficiency - associated recurrent lower extremity venous thrombosis.

D. Diagnosis

This is an area of controversy. A negative perfusion lung scan rules out PE. A high index of suspicion and a high likelihood scan rules in PE. A high clinical suspicion and a positive noninvasive test for deep venous thrombosis of lower extremities calls for treatment. If the clinical suspicion and the lung scan results are divergent, a pulmonary anteriogram may be indicated. Lung scans will remain positive for about one week on heparin. If lung scanning is not immediately available and there are no contra-indications, heparin can be begun pending studies.

E. Treatment

1. Heparin

a. Start heparin 2-3 days before Coumadin to avoid Coumadin skin necrosis in patients with homozygous protein C deficiency.

b. Heparin induced thrombocytopenia. Mild reduction of platelets to around 100,000 on day 7-10. Usually asymptomatic, no bleeding. Direct effect of heparin on platelet. Future heparin not contraindicated. Will be less likely to occur with highly purified heparin highly specific for antithrombin III.

c. Heparin induced thrombosis, "white clot syndrome". Precipitous reduction in platelet count. Associated with deep venous and arterial thrombosis due to in vivo platelet aggregation, may have associated severe morbidity. Autoimmune with antibodies to platelet-heparin complex. Heparin contraindicated.

2. Coumadin

   a. Teratogenic. Many drug-drug interactions, monitor patient when adding new drugs. Heparin is generally safer than Coumadin which is safer than thrombolytics.

   b. Increased Protime with Coumadin:

   > Many antibiotics
   > Allopurinol
   > Acetaminophen
   > Nonsteroidals
   > Quinine and quinidine
   > Sulfonamides
   > Anabolic steroids
   > Lovastatin

   c. Decreased Protime with Coumadin

   > Corticosteroids
   > Barbiturates
   > Griseofulvin
   > Oral contraceptives
   > Cholestyramine

3. Thrombolytics

   a. Must be used with care. Exclusions: Recent CVA, surgery, neurosurgery, post-partum, bleeding ulcer, bleeding diathesis.

4. Embolectomy

   a. Reserved for dire situations, not usually successful.

5. Vena cava ligation, plication, vena cava filter

   a. These are really measures to prevent further emboli. They are appropriate in the patient with definite emboli who has contraindications to anticoagulation such as active GI bleeding, bleeding diathesis, hemorrhagic CVA.

F. Prophylaxis

   1. Candidates

      a. Hospitalized patient at bed rest to include congestive heart failure, MI, pneumonia, thrombotic CVA.

      b. Pre-op patients - gynecologic, abdominal, orthopedic.

   2. Regimens

      a. Low dose subcutaneous 5000 u heparin q 8-12 hours.

      b. This regimen does not work for patients going to hip replacement; they require low dose Coumadin, occasionally aspirin.

      c. The PTT should not be extended with this regimen. However, elderly frail patients, especially "little old ladies" are at risk to bleed on low dose heparin.

      d. If patients develop GI or urinary tract bleeding on anticoagulation, look for an underlying cause (tumor, polyp).

V. **PNEUMONIA**

Covered in section on infectious diseases. Very important!

VI. <u>INTERSTITIAL LUNG DISEASES</u>

A. Inflammation ("Alveolitis")

1. Normal lung

a. 80 Inflammatory cells per alveolus: macrophages (90%), lymphocytes (mainly T), rare PMN.

b. IG's; IgG> IgA>> IgM

c. Complement, antioxidants, antiproteases.

2. Interstitial lung disease (ILD)

a. Increased numbers cells

b. Patterns:

1. macrophage - dominant alveolitis

2. lymphocyte - macrophage alveolitis

subcategory T helper cell - macrophage alveolitis in granulomatous disease: sarcoidosis and berylliosis

3. neutrophil - macrophage alveolitis

B. ILD Secondary to Inhaled Inorganic Dusts

1. Asbestos related disorders

a. Asbestos bodies, fibers

1. Found in most populations studied

2. Requires large biopsies, best done at autopsy

3. Increased numbers in urban populations

4. Fibers in air, drinking water

5. Body's defense mechanisms coat fibers with iron ("ferruginous body")

6. In association with diffuse fibrosis, they confirm the diagnosis of asbestosis

b. Effusions

    1. Occur early in exposure

    2. Usually resolve spontaneously

c. Pleural plaques

    1. Commonly along diaphragm

    2. Best seen with CT

    3. Not associated with disease

d. Small airways disease

    1. Caused by many mineral dusts including asbestos, and most commonly by cigarette smoke.

    2. Does not cause clinical disease.

    3. Detectable by pulmonary function testing FEF 25-75.

    4. Pathologically mineral dust induced small airways disease causes fibrosis of <u>respiratory</u> bronchioles.

    5. Pathologically cigarette smoke induced small airways disease causes fibrosis of <u>membranous</u> bronchioles.

    6. This lesion is different from the <u>diffuse</u> peribronchiolar fibrosis of asbestosis.

e. Industrial bronchitis

    1. Excess mucus production in large airways

    2. Nonspecific reaction to irritation by many dusts and fumes, including asbestos

    3. Minor functional consequences when investigated in coal miners

f. Asbestosis

    1. Symptom: dyspnea

    2. Latency: 20+ years

    3. Exposure: high intensity jobs with repeated exposure to moderate to high levels of fibers

    4. Physical exam: rales, clubbing

    5. CXR: basilar fibrosis

    6. PFT's: restriction (commonly mixed due to high prevalence of COPD)

    7. Pathology: peribronchiolar fibrosis with asbestos bodies. No emphysema

g. Mesothelioma

    1. Fiber type

        a. low risk with serpentine (chrysotile)

        b. high risk with amphibole (crocidolite)

    2. No relation to cigarette smoking

    3. Despite one fiber theory of causation, statistically dose related

h. Lung cancer

    1. All cell types, all lobes

    2. Marked synergism with cigarette smoke; very rare in nonsmokers

    3. More common in patients with underlying asbestosis

    4. Jobs: insulators, shipyard workers, plumbers, construction workers, asbestos abatement workers, textile workers, miners and millers

2. Silicosis

a. Latency: rarely five years to decades

    b. Nodular form

        1. Simple - Small parenchymal lesions, primarily upper lobes, composed of whorled hyalinized collagen surrounded by reticulum and fibroblasts

            No symptoms, normal PFT's

        2. Complicated - progressive massive fibrosis. Nodules > 1 cm, PFT's: decreased VC, TLC, DLCO, pO2

    c. Silicoproteinosis - rare form after intense exposure. Alveolar filling similar to alveolar proteinosis. Severe volume restriction, progressive hypoxia and rapid death.

  3. Coal workers' pneumoconiosis (Black Lung)

    a. Pigmented macrophages around respiratory bronchioles; focal emphysema, increased reticulin and collagen

    b. CXR similar to silicosis

        1. Simple - no symptoms

        2. Progressive massive fibrosis - severe PFT abnormalities and melanoptysis

    c. Risk factors: cumulative dust exposure, quartz, immunologic factors, infectious agents

  4. Berylliosis

    a. resembles sarcoidosis (see below)

C. ILD Secondary to Inhaled Organic Dusts

  1. "Hypersensitivity pneumonitis" OR

     "Extrinsic allergic alveolitis"

     Prototype: Farmer's lung due to Micropolyspora, Thermophilic Actinomyces, Aspergillus.

2. History is paramount!

    a. Acute form:

       Cough, fever, chills, malaise

       Dyspnea 6-8 hours post exposure, symptoms clear up over few days

    b. Subacute form:

       Insidious cough and dyspnea

       May require hospitalization

       May occur after acute form if antigen not removed

       Work up is individualized

       Challenge tests with suspected antigen, serum precipitins, open lung biopsy may be done.

       Improvement on removal from workplace is helpful in diagnosis, along with clearing of chest x-ray.

3. Pathogenesis

    a. Immediate IgE mediated response to aerosolized antigen.

    b. Delayed complex response involving multiple immune components

    c. Only a few of the exposed population ever develop the disorder; may be a problem of immune suppression

4. Histology

    a. Acute phase does not come to biopsy

    b. Subacute and chronic phases: granulomatous involvement of central portion of lobule with bronchiolitis and alveolitis

D. ILD Secondary to Drugs

1. Bleomycin

2. Methotrexate

3. Nitrofurantoin

4. Amiodarone

5. Phenytoin

6. Gold

7. Allopurinol

E. ILD of Unknown Etiology

1. Connective tissue disorders

2. Idiopathic pulmonary fibrosis

3. Vasculitis

4. Inherited

5. With other organ system disease

6. Sarcoidosis

   a. Clinical findings

      1. Patients with sarcoid are usually asymptomatic.

      Affects many organs, but most commonly the lung.

      2. Perihilar and R paratracheal nodes ("potato nodes"), interstitial infiltrates, pulmonary fibrosis.

      3. Facial rash "lupus pernio" (lacy reticular rash), erythema nodosum over shins, skin plaques.

      4. Liver granulomas, muscle tenderness and elevated CPK.

      5. Uveoparotid fever (Heerfordt's Syndrome) with uveitis and salivary gland involvement similar to sicca syndrome; facial nerve palsy.

      6. Large joint involvement.

      7. Neurohypophysis involvement with diabetes insipidus; Mononeuritis multiplex or poly-neuropathy.

      8. Heart involvement with conduction abnor-malities.

b. Pathophysiology

      1. Not completely understood.

      2. Inciting agent not known.

      3. Recruitment of inflammatory cells by T4 cells.

      4. Polyclonal gammopathy produced by B cells.

      5. Production of granulomata in affected organs (usually asymptomatic).

c. Lab findings

      1. Depend on organ system involved.

      2. Polyclonal gammopathy common.

      3. Hypercalcemia common.

            a. Overabsorption of calcium from gut.

            b. Granulomas produce Vitamin D.

            c. May cause renal disease.

      4. Elevated serum angiotensin converting enzyme. Along with gallium scan, has been used in diagnosis.

d. Diagnosis

      1. Classic presentation. Young person aged 20-40, asymptomatic, with bilaterally sym-metric hilar or paratracheal adenopathy.

      2. Skin biopsy, if lesions.

3. Transbronchial lung biopsy.

    a. + 60% even if negative CXR.

    b. + 90% if parenchymal lesions on CXR.

4. Blind muscle or liver biopsy can show non-caseating granulomata.

5. Exclude specific organisms by special stains and cultures.

6. Kveim test rarely used. (An antigen made from tissue of sarcoid patients and injected intradermally causing a very delayed (weeks) skin response in sarcoid patients).

  e. Treatment

1. None may be required if asymptomatic.

2. Obtain baseline pulmonary functions and use abnormal decreased vital capacity and diffusing capacity to follow treatment.

3. Treat pulmonary, eye and CNS symptoms with steroids. Taper when possible.

  f. Prognosis

1. Generally good. May spontaneously regress.

2. Rarely progresses to pulmonary fibrosis and respiratory insufficiency.

F. Therapy of ILD

1. Remove patient from offending agent!

    May involve career change, disability proceedings, lawyers, paperwork

2. Suppress alveolitis

  a. Corticosteroids

1. Prednisone 1 mg/kg/d for 1-2 months, taper over 2-3 months to maintenance dose of 0.25 mg/kg/d

        2. Dosed once daily

    a. Corticosteroids

    b. Cytotoxics

    c. Assessment of response

       Symptoms may not abate since severely damaged alveoli are lost.

    d. Treat intercurrent infections

    e. Bronchodilators

    f. Oxygen

G. Occupational Asthma

  1. Definition

    Disorder of function characterized by reversible airways obstruction.

  2. Parkes' patterns of workplace exposure

    a. Deterioration during workday with improvement on leaving.

    b. Deterioration during work week with improvement on weekend.

    c. Progressive deterioration week by week where intervening weekend not sufficient for symptom resolution.

    d. Maximum deterioration in first day of work week with later recovery.

3. Etiologies

Chemicals	Grain and Flour
Formalin	Wheat
Fluorine	Flour
Drugs	Hops
Isocyanates	Insects
Metals	Animals and Birds
Platinum	Rodents
Nickel	Feathers
Wood Dust	
Fungi	
Mushroom spores	

4. Pathology

a. Not well studied

b. Assumed to be similar to allergic asthma with normal lung parenchyma and inflammatory airway changes.

VII. **LUNG ABSCESS**

Due to destruction of lung parenchyma by pyogenic organism.

A. Symptoms

Malaise, cough, fever, putrid sputum. Consider in predisposed patient (see below) who doesn't improve with usual treatment of pneumonia.

B. Physical findings

Early: may look like pneumonia patients, though they "fail to thrive" with treatment, look chronically ill, hectic fever.

Late: clubbing, weight loss.

C. High risk patients

Poor dentition
Aspiration
Alcoholism
Altered consciousness
Malignancy
Right-sided endocarditis
Foreign body

D. Diagnosis

CXR may show air fluid level. CT may show cavity. Bronchoscopy may help with diagnosis and therapy by promoting drainage.

E. Treatment

Penicillin, clindamycin for likely anaerobes. Physical therapy, bronchoscopy to promote drainage, CT directed chest tube placement for drainage, occasional instillation of antibiotics.

VIII. **BRONCHIECTASIS**

A. Symptoms

Copious sputum, frequent infections, posterior basilar segments and R middle lobe commonly involved due to gravity and lack of good drainage.

B. Diagnosis

CXR, CT Scan, <u>bronchography</u> (can have serious complications).

C. High risk patients

Patients with congenital abnormalities of bronchi. Patients with congenital or acquired <u>hypogamma-globulinemia</u>, cystic fibrosis, alpha-1-antitrypsin deficiency.

D. Treatment

Antimicrobials, physical therapy to promote drainage, rarely surgery as the process tends not to be confined.

IX. **TUBERCULOSIS**

A. Primary infection

Usually asymptomatic infection of nonimmune person in middle or lower lobe, may involve hilar nodes. Acquired by contact with aerosol from patient with cavitary disease. Usual inflammatory response occurs with later caseous necrosis, calcification and scarring of pulmonary parenchyma and node, together called Ghon complex. The earliest phase may be associated with hematogenous spread, causing miliary TB and meningitis. The organisms remain dormant in the scar and may be slowly inactivated. The macrophage is the cell capable of containing the organism. Delayed hyper- sensitivity (positive skin test) occurs temporally with containment of the organism.

B. Latency

The bugs may remain dormant for the remainder of the patient's life. Inactive lesions can contain viable bacilli.

C. Reactivation

Usual mechanism for development of active TB in adult. Dormant foci in upper lobes, acquired at time of hematogenous dissemination of primary infection, become active. Symptoms are usually gradual with fatigue, fever, cough, night sweats, weight loss, hemoptysis.

D. Diagnosis

1. Suspect in high risk groups.

2. Skin test

   Intermediate strength, 5 tuberculin units, 0.1 cc given intradermally (Mantoux) with 10 mm of induration is positive. If a 250 unit 2nd strength test is negative, active TB is <u>highly</u> unlikely. Anergy batteries helpful to prove a negative is really negative.

3. Get sputums for AFB smear and culture.

4. Cavitary disease associated with positive smears. Consider a patient infectious until smear negative.

E. Treatment

1. Active disease, compliant patient.

    a. Long course (in past)

        INH, ethambutol for 1 1/2 - 2 years with rifampin or streptomycin initial supplements for 1 - 2 months.

    b. Short course

        INH and rifampin for 9 months; 3rd drug at outset decreases chance of drug resistance; 3rd drug may shorten to 6 months.

    c. Active disease, non-compliant patient.

        1. Intermittent twice weekly supervised 4 drug regimen with INH, ethambutol, rifampin, streptomycin. Given after 1st 2 months of daily therapy.

    d. Trend has been to short course therapy.

    e. For prophylaxis

        1. In close contacts with negative skin tests.

        2. For known skin test converters.

        3. For skin test positive patients who become immunosuppressed.

        4. INH 300 mg. daily X 1 yr. Main side effect is hepatitis.

    f. Drug resistance

        1. Becoming more of a problem in the 90's.

        2. Multiple drugs are used in combination to prevent drug resistance.

        3. Non-compliance, increased numbers of infected Asians and Hispanics will increase drug resistance.

F. Extrapulmonary TB

1. CNS

    a. Inflammation at base of brain.

    b. Looks like other causes of chronic meningitis
        with CSF lymphocytes, increased protein,
        decreased glucose.

2. Lymphadenitis

    a. Most common extrapulmonary manifestation
        world-wide.

    b. If cervical, called scrofula. May be due to
        other than M TB.

3. Pericarditis

    a. Can be a cause of acute and chronic
        pericarditis leading to constrictive
        pericarditis.

    b. Diagnosis may be difficult due to commonly
        negative skin test, paucity of organisms in
        fluid and its nonspecificity, lack of TB
        elsewhere in body.

    c. Empiric therapy when there is a high index of
        suspicion is justified.

4. Genitourinary

    a. Hematogenous spread, renal abscesses, ureteral
        scarring, hydronephrosis. Produces "sterile
        pyuria" with usual cultures.

    b. Tuberculous cystitis produces a small, scarred
        bladder causing dysuria and frequency.

    c. Genital

        1. Chronic draining scrotal tract and
            prostatitis in males.

        2. Pelvic inflammatory disease in females.

        3. Sterility.

    d.   Peritonitis

        1.   Commonly a complication of genital TB.

        2.   Painless ascites.

        3.   Laparoscopy may be helpful to diagnose.

5.   Osseous

    a.   Pott's disease: Gibbus (hump) deformity <u>thoracic</u> and <u>lumbar</u> spine.

    b.   Infection begins in disk space (<u>unlike cancer</u> which generally does not cross disk space) and spreads to contiguous vertebrae.

    c.   Paravertebral mass seen on x-ray.

6.   Joints

    a.   Chronic monoarticular arthritis of hips and knees.

    b.   Seen with atypicals in HIV patients.

G.   Atypicals

1.   Mycobacterium avium-intracellulare complex most common.

2.   A major problem in AIDS patients.

3.   Cause extrapulmonary disease: wasting syndrome, intestinal, joints; can be grown from blood.

4.   Resistant organisms may require 5 or more drugs, often with considerable toxicity.

5.   The disease in AIDS is chronic and requires lifelong therapy.

6.   Other clinical settings

    a.   Historically: infected sternum after CABG when contaminated bone wax used.

    b.   COPD patient with cultured atypicals in sputum; need evidence of cavity or infiltrate to consider pathogenic and treat.

7. Not transmitted person-to-person; acquired from environment.

H. High Risk Patients

1. Alcoholics

2. Malnourished (gastrectomy)

3. AIDS/HIV, injection drug users, patients in confinement such as prisons. Occurs earlier in course in HIV disease than atypicals; more virulent.

4. Blacks, Eskimos

5. Immunosuppressed, on chemotherapy or dialysis, steroids, malnourished.

6. Crowding

X. PULMONARY HYPERTENSION

Prototype: Primary Pulmonary Hypertension

A. Early symptoms

1. Vague symptoms, increased fatigue, hard to diagnose. Late symptoms: chest pains, breathlessness, syncope.

2. Associated with sudden death, especially during invasive procedures, unknown reasons.

B. Physical exam

1. R ventricular lift along left sternal border, enlarged "a" waves in jugular pulse, loud P2, ejection click, right heart S4.

2. Late clubbing of fingers, hepatomegaly, S3.

C. Studies

1. CXR shows enlarged pulmonary arteries with "pruning" of peripheral vessels, cardiomegaly.

2. EKG shows R ventricular hypertrophy.

3. Lung scan useful to exclude pulmonary emboli.

    4. Cardiac catheterization shows pulmonary arterial hypertension with normal pulmonary wedge pressure and near normal cardiac output.

D. At Risk

    1. Young women of reproductive age.

    2. Familiar cases occur.

    3. Epidemic cases occurred after use of anorectic agent Aminorex in Europe.

E. Pathogenesis

    1. Unknown but obliteration of small pulmonary arteries occurs in concentric fashion (as opposed to recurrent pulmonary emboli where eccentric fibroelastosis occurs). Theories of persistent fetal pulmonary vascular bed, sustained vasoconstriction, autoimmune.

F. Treatment

    1. Vasodilators

       Hydralazine, Nifedipine, Prostacyclin

    2. Coumadin (new)

    3. Oxygen

    4. Heart-lung transplant

G. Prognosis

    1. Very poor, usually death within few years.

H. Differential Diagnoses to Rule-Out

    1. Recurrent pulmonary emboli

    2. Interstitial lung diseases

       a. Connective tissue diseases

       b. Asbestosis

       c. Sarcoidosis

    3. Veno-occlusive disease

XI. DISRUPTIONS OF THE MECHANICS OF VENTILATION

A. Pneumothorax

1. Symptoms

   Sudden dyspnea, sudden pleurisy. Patients may be asymptomatic at rest but have severe exertional dyspnea.

2. Physical findings

   Tachypnea, tachycardia, decreased or absent breath sounds on ipsilateral side.

3. Etiologies

   a. Trauma

   b. Spontaneous, young men, commonly right-sided

   c. Ruptured bleb in bullous emphysema

   d. Rib fracture

   e. PEEP on ventilator

   f. Catamenial (menstruating women with endometriosis)

   g. Eosinophilic granuloma

   h. Iatrogenic from subclavian stick

4. Treatment

   a. Observe if < 30% and patient tolerating.

   b. Chest tube if patient sick or large pneumothorax.

B. Flail Chest: Seen with multiple rib fractures

C. Atelectasis

1. common post operatively

2. may be secondary to obstruction of bronchus

XII. <u>QUESTIONS</u>

1. In pulmonary function testing, a decreased FEV-1 (forced expiratory volume in one second) is most indicative of

   a. an obstructive lung disease
   b. a restrictive lung disease

2. Hypoxemia derives largely from the following pulmonary disorder

   a. right to left shunt
   b. alveolar hypoventilation
   c. diffusion abnormality
   d. all of the above

3. Hypoventilation can be caused by

   a. hypothyroidism
   b. metabolic alkalosis
   c. sedatives
   d. hypophosphatemia
   e. all of the above

4. The most common pathogen found in the sputum of bronchitics is

   a. Pneumococcus
   b. Haemophilus influenza
   c. Branhamella (Moraxella) catarrhalis
   d. all of the above

5. Important associations with asthmatics include

   a. aspirin sensitivity or allergy
   b. history of nasal polyps
   c. sinusitis
   d. all of the above

6. The gold standard for the definitive diagnosis of a pulmonary embolus is

    a. a VQ scan
    b. pulmonary angiography
    c. chest x-ray
    d. CAT scan of the chest

7. The leading cause of exudative pleural effusions is

    a. cancer
    b. congestive heart failure
    c. nephrotic syndrome
    d. infections

8. A common setting for aspiration pneumonia is

    a. depressed mental status
    b. nasogastric tube
    c. seizure
    d. drunkenness
    e. all of the above

9. The differential diagnosis of hemoptysis may include

    a. cancer
    b. bronchiectasis
    c. tuberculosis
    d. lung abscess
    e. pulmonary infarction
    f. all of the above

10. Cor pulmonale is a term applied to right ventricular enlargement secondary to pulmonary hypertension.

    _____ True   _____ False

11. An increased A-a gradient represents

    a. hypoxemia
    b. hypercapnia
    c. pneumonia
    d. shunting
    e. metabolic alkalosis

12. A 36-year-old white female presents with pleurisy, dyspnea, and ABG's showing hypoxemia and respiratory alkalosis. You want to ask about all EXCEPT

    a. use of oral contraceptives
    b. prior similar episodes
    c. traveler's diarrhea
    d. pregnancy
    e. cross country travel by auto

13. Asbestosis shows which one of the following on chest x-ray?

    a. bilateral upper lobe infiltrates
    b. bilateral lower lobe infiltrates
    c. bilateral upper lobe fibrosis
    d. bilateral upper lobe cavities
    e. bilateral lower lobe cavities

14. Farmer's lung is the prototype of

    a. connective tissue lung disease
    b. hereditary lung disease
    c. nosocomial lung disease
    d. hypersensitivity lung disease
    e. infectious lung disease

15. All except one of the following are problematic in patients with severe COPD

    a. Nocardia
    b. mycobacterium kansasii
    c. typical tuberculosis
    d. HIV
    e. mycobacterium avium-intracellulare

16. The treatment of choice for allergic asthma is

    a. oral beta-2 bronchodilators
    b. oral theophylline
    c. inhaled steroids
    d. oral steroids
    e. parenteral steroids

17. Chronic bronchitics most often complain of

    a. chest pains, substernal
    b. chest pains, pleuritic
    c. cough and sputum
    d. air hunger
    e. weight loss

18. Patient with emphysema most often complain of

    a. chest pains, substernal
    b. fever and sputum
    c. cough and sputum
    d. dyspnea
    e. weight loss

19. Nicotine addiction is as powerful an addiction as heroin.

    _____ True   _____ False

20. Indications for oxygen include all EXCEPT

    a. hypoxemia with pO2 below 55
    b. desaturation with exercise
    c. secondary polycythemia
    d. cor pulmonale
    e. FEV1 below 1.9 liters

21. Erythromycin as initial outpatient therapy for community-acquired pneumonia is a good choice because of its effectiveness against

    a. pneumococcus
    b. mycoplasma
    c. Legionnaire's disease
    d. all of the above

22. One judges the quality of a sputum smear by

    a. numbers of gram-positive bacteria per high-powered field
    b. numbers of gram-negative bacteria
    c. presence of eosinophilic staining mucus
    d. presence of leukocytes and absence of squamous epithelial cells

23. The choice of empiric antibiotic therapy in a 65-year-old male with an infiltrate depends upon all but

    a. presence of underlying COPD
    b. acquisition of pneumonia in community or hospital
    c. presence of underlying lung abscess
    d. creatinine
    e. PO2

XIII. ANSWERS

  1. a

  2. d

  3. e

  4. d

  5. d

  6. b

  7. a

  8. e

  9. f

10. True

11. d

12. c

13. b

14. d

15. d

16. c

17. c

18. d

19. True

20. e

21. d

22. d

23. e

CHAPTER 3: RENAL DISEASE

I. **ACUTE TUBULAR NECROSIS**

A. Symptoms

    1. Fatigue, weakness, anorexia.

    2. Decreased urine output.

B. Signs

    1. Hypertension, evidence of fluid retention (pedal edema, increased neck veins, rales).

    2. Oliguria.

    3. Abnormal urine: pigmented cellular casts and renal tubular epithelial cells.,

    4. Urine sodium is high, usually > 40 meg/L.

C. At Risk Patients

    1. Hypotension

    2. Sepsis

    3. Cardiogenic shock

    4. Surgery, especially with ischemia to kidneys from cross clamping aorta

    5. Iodinated contrast

    6. Drugs

D. Clinical Course (two types)

1. Oliguric (> 50% of patients).

    a. These patients suffer an insult, usually hypotension, during which time urine flow drops. At this point, hydration, mannitol, loop diuretics may reverse. <u>Oliguria</u> (400 - 800 cc/d) then develops. <u>Anuria</u> (< 400 cc/d) uncommon (Think obstruction).

    b. Creatinine and BUN rise and are roughly 1:10 ratio, indicating <u>renal</u> damage! Pre-renal and post-renal problems have a relatively higher BUN.

    c. K+ increases and CO_2 decreases.

    d. Indications for dialysis:

        Fluid retention   (Not controlled
        Hyperkalemia   by medical means)
        Acidosis

    e. Oliguria commonly persists 10-14 days. Urine flow increases, but metabolic abnormalities may not resolve immediately.

    f. High mortality (30-60%). Most usually no permanent clinical renal damage.

    g. Oliguric phase may be prolonged (weeks) in elderly patients with vascular disease.

2. Nonoliguric - Patient continues to make urine. Though metabolic problems continue, fluid overload is not a problem.

3. Management of ATN

    a. Remove any nephrotoxins (especially drugs).

    b. Restrict fluid; replace what is lost plus insensible loss.

    c. Restrict dietary protein; may need parenteral hyperalimentation with amino acid solution.

    d. Expect weight loss up to 1 lb. per day.

e. Protect stomach with H2 blockers and sucralfate (high incidence of GI bleed).

f. Hyperphosphatemia can be treated with phosphate binding antacids (Amphojel). Avoid magnesium containing antacids (most of the commonly used preps).

g. Treat hyperkalemia with Kayexelate.

h. Hypocalcemia usually does not require treatment.

i. Treat any infection with non-nephrotoxic drugs.

j. Acidosis generally doesn't require treatment until severe (bicarb - 10).

k. Expect anemia, though may be well tolerated. Transfusion may be necessary. Mild bleeding tendency may occur.

l. Expect hypertension, usually secondary to volume overload.

m. Prevent ATN if possible.

1. Check blood levels of commonly used nephrotoxic drugs such as aminoglycosides and vancomycin.

2. Avoid iodinated contrast in patients with borderline renal function (creat > 1.7), diabetics, myeloma patients, elderly with vascular disease.

3. If absolutely necessary to give contrast, hydrate well and use mannitol pre-contrast.

II. **PRE-RENAL AZOTEMIA**

A. Suspect in patients who are dehydrated, have congestive heart failure, end stage liver disease, infections (pneumonia, sepsis).

B. BUN is relatively much higher than creatinine (>10:1).

C. Urine contains hyaline casts, few formed elements.

D. Urine sodium is low, usually < 10 meg/L.

III. POST-RENAL AZOTEMIA

A. Suspect in patients with decreased urine output, rising BUN and creatinine (ratio > 10:1) who have:

1. Prostate hypertrophy or cancer.

2. Neurogenic bladder (paraplegics, diabetics, patients with multiple sclerosis, etc.).

3. Cervical cancer (utereral obstruction due to tumor).

4. Single kidney either anatomically or functionally whose lone ureter is vulnerable to obstruction. (Remember unilateral ureteral obstruction in a patient with two functioning kidneys does not cause renal failure).

5. Urethral strictures.

This can be a chronic problem usually due to congenital urethral valves or past history of gonorrhea.

6. Prior surgery on the urinary tract. Diverting procedures, ureterostomy.

7. History of reflux of urine from bladder into ureters; congenital or acquired uretero- pelvic narrowing.

8. Foley catheter. It may be positioned incorrectly.

9. Phimosis

10. Use of anticholinergic drugs, pain medications, decongestants.

B. Document obstruction with an ultrasound, not an IVP. (Would cause further renal failure due to contrast.)

Expect to see bilateral hydronephrosis in patient with two functioning kidneys.

C. After above, do something to relieve obstruction! (place or replace Foley, ureteral stents, nephrostomy tube, remove stone, etc.)

D. This is a very treatable condition. Don't miss it!!

IV. __HEMATURIA__

A. __Red Cell__ Hematuria

1. Needs to be evaluated always.

2. Urethral - uncommon except for iatrogenic, due to Foley trauma.

3. Bladder

   a. Hemorrhagic cystitis common, also bacterial infections, cyclophosphamide.

   b. If aseptic, think of interstitial cystitis in young to middle age females.

   c. If chronic, need to exclude bladder tumors, polyps, diverticuli.

4. Prostate

   a. Common with BPH, after prostate biopsy.

   b. Need cystoscopy to diagnose.

5. Ureteral

   a. Most often due to stone.

   b. Calcium oxalate will show on KUB, uric acid will not.

6. Kidney

   a. Need to exclude tumor, hematoma, trauma.

   b. Seen with sickle cell trait, IgA nephropathy, TB.

7. Pelvis

   a. Seen after trauma with pelvic bone fracture.

8. Anticoagulation

Bleeding site(s) may not be localized with our usual tests.

9. Menstrual

Don't chase this. Ask your patient.

B. Red Cell <u>Cast</u> Hematuria

1. Glomerulonephritis

Disease	Pathology
Post streptococcal GN	<u>Lumpy</u> deposits of IgG in mesangium, circulating immune complexes.
Rapidly progressive GN (subset Goodpasture's)	<u>Crescentic</u> glomerulonephritis with extensive extra-capillary proliferation.
Nephrotic syndrome	
a. Subset minimal change disease (good prognosis)	EM findings of diffuse epithelial <u>foot process</u> effacement or fusion.
b. Subset focal glomerulosclerosis	<u>Sclerosis</u> and hyalinization of some but not all glomeruli
c. Subset membranous glomerulopathy	Irregular IgG on <u>subepithelial</u> aspect of glomerular capillary wall of all glomeruli.
d. Subset membranoproliferative glomerulonephritis.	Proliferation of mesangial cells.

Renal biopsies are uncommonly done but may be necessary to differentiate the above. Post-streptococcal disease can be diagnosed by ASO titer or streptozyme in the proper clinical setting.

2. Vasculitis

C. Hemoglobinuria

   1. Acute hemolysis, rapid, intravascular.

   2. Paroxysmal nocturnal hemoglobinuria

   3. Positive dipstick for blood, no RBC's

D. Myoglobin "Hematuria"

   1. Positive dipstick for blood, no RBC's.

   2. Check urine for myoglobin.

   3. Seen after crush injury to muscle, prolonged time in one position, some infections.

V. PYURIA

A. Urethritis

   1. Gonorrhea, non-gonococcal, Reiter's

B. Cystitis

   1. Will usually have accompanying dysuria, frequency.

   2. May be asymptomatic after instrumentation or with Foley.

C. Interstitial Renal Disease

   1. Acute interstitial nephritis

      a. Drug induced

         1. NSAID's, penicillin, sulfonamides, allopurinol

         2. Captopril, gold, diuretics

      b. Eosinophils in tissue, urine, blood.

      c. Hematuria, fever, renal failure.

   2. Toxins

      a. Heavy metals

      b. Solvents, hydrocarbons

3. Infections (TB)

4. Chronic interstitial nephritis

   a. Analgesic nephropathy (acetaminophen, phenacetin)

   b. Progression of acute processes

D. Pyelonephritis, Acute

1. Accompanying fever, flank pain, abdominal pain, nausea.

2. May have symptoms of cystitis.

3. Risk factors: pregnancy, females, diabetics, abnormal urinary anatomy.

VI. **PROTEINURIA**

A. Must work up if > 1+ on dipstick, no obvious infection.

B. Do protein electrophoresis to separate albumin and the various globulin fractions (can determine monoclonal gammopathy seen with myeloma).

C. Albuminuria

1. Seen with glomerular lesions.

2. Nephrotic syndrome.

   a. Greater than 3.5g/24 hours.

   b. Creatinine may be normal.

   c. Seen with diabetes, gold, membranous glomerulonephritis, lung cancer, Hodgkin's.

   d. Clinical edema.

   e. Associated hyperlipidemia.

D. Gamma Globulinuria (Bence Jones proteinuria).

1. Light chains excreted in myeloma, Waldenstrom's, light chain disease, amyloid.

2. May be monoclonal kappa or lambda; both are toxic to kidney tubules but the latter more so ("lethal lambda").

3. Myeloma kidney: renal failure due to toxic light chains; effect of hypercalcemia (from bony lesions) on tubule to prevent water reabsorption (polyuria) leading to dehydration; coexisting amyloid causing glomerular disease. Any further insult (IVP dye, aminoglycoside, hypotension) may lead to irreversible renal failure.

VII. <u>CHRONIC RENAL INSUFFICIENCY/FAILURE</u>

A. Whatever the initiating event, chronic renal failure presents a similar clinical picture of gradual and irreversible nephron loss.

B. Urine sediment contains <u>broad</u> casts, reflecting compensatory dilatation of surviving nephrons.

C. Management

1. Prevent dehydration.

2. Treat hypertension.

3. Avoid nephrotoxins.

4. Treat UTI's.

5. Use phosphate binding antacids. Avoid magnesium antacids.

6. Treat anemia with erythropoietin.

7. Treat acidosis with bicarbonate/citrate solutions (Shohl's).

8. Use calcium supplements.

9. Correct dosing of medication in renal failure/use of drugs excreted by liver.

10. Special care for dialysis patients

a. Vitamin supplements.

b. Care of venous access or peritoneal catheter.

    c. High index of suspicion for infection, sepsis.

VIII. HEREDITARY RENAL DISEASES

A. With Associated Sensorineural **Deafness**: Alport's Syndrome

    1. Males more often and more severely affected, associated with X chromosome

    2. Recurrent hematuria, renal failure.

B. With **Cutaneous** Lesions: Fabry's disease

    1. X-linked, accumulation of sphingolipids.

    2. Purple macules.

C. With **Nephrolithiasis**

    1. Medullary sponge kidney:

        a. Autosomal dominant.

        b. Diagnose by IVP showing dilated cystic terminal collecting ducts, calcifications, calcium oxalate stones.

        c. Renal failure is rare.

    2. Hyperoxaluria: autosomal recessive, irreversible renal failure before age 20.

D. With **Cysts**: Polycystic kidney disease

    1. Associated liver and pancreas cysts.

    2. Large palpable kidneys.

    3. Maintained hemoglobin despite renal failure.

    4. Autosomal dominant. Hematuria, infection, stones.

E. With **Acidosis**

    1. Distal type 1 renal tubular acidosis:

        a. Autosomal dominant; bone disease (rickets in children, osteomalacia in adults) due to renal hypercalciuria.

b. Inability to acidify urine less than pH 5.5., hyperchloremic acidosis.

c. Treat with bicarbonate and citrate.

2. Proximal type 2 renal tubular acidosis:

a. Due to bicarbonate wasting.

b. Multiple modes of inheritance.

c. Must replace potassium.

F. With disorders of amino acid transport

1. Cystinuria: cystine is insoluble and causes stones, autosomal recessive.

2. Fanconi syndrome:

a. Proximal tubule transport defects of water, sodium, potassium along with amino acids, monosaccharides.

b. Suspect with glycosuria in the face of normal blood sugar.

c. Autosomal recessive, renal failure rare.

IX. STONE DISEASE

Disease	Stone	Treatment
Hyperparathyroidism	Calcium	Fluids and remove adenoma
Hypercalciuria	Calcium	Thiazides
Hyperuricosuria	Calcium & Uric Acid	Allopurinol
Intestinal hyper-oxaluria (from ileal disease or absence)	Calcium	Cholestyramine, Oxalate, supplemental calcium.
Gout	Uric Acid	Allopurinol
UTI, recurrent and chronic	Struvite	Antibiotics, remove stones.

X. DISORDERS OF ACID BASE AND ELECTROLYTES

A. Hyperchloremic Acidosis

Renal Tubular acidosis - see prior discussion.

1. RTA type 1 "classic distal" can be seen in paint sniffers due to toluene. Hypokalemia can be severe (1.6) with resulting extreme muscle weakness (paralysis). Acidosis is also severe but usually amenable to treatment with fluids and bicarbonate.

2. Causes of Distal "classic" type I RTA

    Genetic
    Many drugs (Amphotericin B, toluene)
    Autoimmune diseases
    Hematologic diseases
    Renal diseases
    Endocrine diseases (hyperparathyroidism)

3. Distal RTA "generalized" is commonly seen in the setting of diabetics with renal insufficiency who take nonsteroidals. They get resultant hyperkalemia. The syndrome is also called hyporeninemic hypoaldosteronism.

4. Causes of Proximal type II RTA

    Genetic
    Idiopathic
    Acetazolamide

Type	K+	Urinary pH	Renal defect
Classic distal RTA type I	decreased	> 5.5	cannot excrete acid distally
Generalized distal RTA type IV	increased	< 5.5	decreased aldosterone effect
Proximal Type II	decreased	< 5.5	wastes bicarbonate proximally

B.   Anion Gap Acidosis

   1.   Diabetic Ketoacidosis

      a.   Diagnosis - Easy.   Look for hyperglycemia, acidosis and serum ketones greater than 1:1 dilution (Less than that can be due to starvation).

      b.   Management - Normal saline and insulin. Add glucose back to intravenous fluids when blood sugar is around 250 mg %.   Watch K+ and replace as acidosis improves.   Watch urine output.

   2.   Nonketotic Hyperosmolar Syndrome.

      a.   Dehydration, lethargy, stupor

      b.   Very high glucose (mean 1000 mg%), no ketones.

      c.   Associated with higher mortality rates than DKA, as patients are usually older with other medical problems.

      d.   Treat with saline initially and insulin drip.

      e.   Frequently iatrogenic from steroids, diuretics, phenytoin.

   3.   Alcoholic Ketoacidosis:

      a.   A disorder of binge drinking, starvation, depletion of glycogen.

      b.   Management - replace glucose, give fluids

   4.   Poisonings

      a.   ethylene glycol (look for oxalate crystals in urine)

      b.   methanol;   may progress to blindness, treat with EtOH

      c.   paraldehyde; this smells strong! Alcoholics may use it for DT's.

C. Metabolic Alkalosis Syndromes

1. "Contraction" alkalosis due to:

   a. NG suction without proper replacement fluids

   b. Vigorous diuretic use

2. Bartter's syndrome (rare, good for exams)

   a. Prominent hypokalemia, no hypertension, no edema, excess renin, excess aldosterone

   b. Defective loop of Henle with inability to reabsorb chloride as primary problem

   c. Autosomal recessive

   d. Looks like diuretic abuse. Also exclude chronic vomiting, diarrhea, laxative abuse, check urinary chloride (greater than 20 mEq/L in Bartter's and diuretic use, less than 20 mEq/L in others)

   e. Excess kinin - prostaglandin production. Treat with nonsteroidals, usually indomethacin and potassium replacement.

3. COPD patient on ventilator.

   a. Usually patient has had CO_2 retention and chronic compensated respiratory acidosis, compensated by urinary retention of bicarbonate.

   b. Then the patient is intubated, ventilated, and the CO_2 is blown off, with resulting metabolic alkalosis.

   c. Avoid over-diuresis, treat with KCl.

D. Hyponatremic Syndromes

1. Syndrome of inappropriate antidiuretic hormone

   a. Symptoms - nausea, confusion, seizures (usually Na < 120)

   b. ADH stimulates adenyl cyclase and cyclic AMP to produce hypertonic urine by

       1. making the collecting duct water permeable, allowing resorption and

       2. increasing NaCl absorption by medullary ascending loop of Henle leading to increased medullary tonicity.

   c. Etiologies

       1. lung disease (pneumonia, fibrosis, mass)

       2. malignancy, especially small cell carcinoma

       3. pain

       4. narcotics

       5. Vincristine, Cyclophosphamide

   d. Diagnose with serum Na low (usually less than 130) and inappropriately concentrated urine without other confounding factors such as hypothyroidism or adrenal insufficiency.

   e. Treatment

       1. Fluid restrict! Use of normal saline usually won't work. Use of hypertonic saline dangerous.

       2. Rapid correction (less than 24 hours) can cause pontine myelinolysis, coma, death. Reports of this in otherwise healthy young women.

       3. Be careful!

2. Fluid overload states

   a. Congestive heart failure

       1. Excess renin, aldosterone.

       2. ACE inhibitors commonly used.

   b. Chronic liver disease

       1. Excess aldosterone.

       2. Aldactone commonly used.

3. Vigorous diuresis is dangerous, as are sudden volume shifts of any kind (paracentesis of large quantities) which can precipitate hepatorenal syndrome and death.

    c. Hypothyroidism

       1. These patients have excess water in tissues and body cavities.

       2. Physical findings of puffiness, periorbital and pretibial edema, pericardial and pleural effusions.

F. Hypercalcemia

1. Symptoms - constipation, lethargy, confusions, muscle weakness

2. Signs - dehydration; signs of underlying disorder

3. Etiologies

Hyperparathyroidism	Immobilization
Hyperthyroidism	Malignancy
Calcium containing antacids	Lytic lesions
Thiazide diuretics	
Osteoclast activating factor	
Dehydration	

G. Hypouricemia

1. Etiologies

Oral contrast agents
SIADH
Hodgkin's disease
Allopurinol
Volume overload

XI. QUESTIONS

1. A 55 year old white male veteran presented with a 3 day history of lethargy and confusion. His appetite has been poor and he had not had a bowel movement in 5 days. Physical examination revealed mild hypotension and profound generalized weakness. His low back and ribs were tender to palpation and movement.

Lab: Hgb 7.8 g/dl, creat 4.0, calcium 16.2, SGOT 45, bilirubin 1.2

The most likely diagnosis is: (one best answer)

a. Hyperparathyroidism
b. Multiple myeloma
c. Milk alkali syndrome
d. Hepatorenal syndrome
e. Calcium oxalate kidney stone

The most urgent aspect of his treatment is institution of: (one best answer)

a. Antibiotics
b. Antipyretics
C. Fluids
d. Antacids
e. Steroids

The reason for his clinical presentation is (multiple true-false):

a. Lack of oral intake
b. Polyuria caused by hypercalcemia
c. Confusion caused by hypercalcemia
d. Decreased oxygen carrying capacity due to anemia
e. Constipation due to hypercalcemia
f. High output heart failure
g. Middle cerebral artery thrombosis

2. An 18 year old white male presented to his physician in early September with tea colored urine and leg swelling. He had been previously healthy except for a sore throat several days earlier, which he had ignored due to rush week activities at his college campus. Several new friends also had been ill.

Exam revealed BP 180/116. P 90, T 98, R 26. Neck veins were slightly distended, throat was clear, PMI slightly displaced to L of mid-clavicular line. Lungs clear, abdomen soft, 1-2+ pitting pretibial edema. Creatinine was 3.2, Hgb 11.9.

You want to personally examine his: (Your attending will say all of these, but choose one)

a. Blood smear
b. Sputum
c. Freshly voided urine
d. Serum protein electrophoresis
e. Chemistry profile

The best explanation for his findings is:

a. Stress due to leaving home
b. Chlamydia pharyngitis sequelae
c. Mycoplasma pharyngitis sequelae
d. Acute post streptococcal glomerulonephritis
e. Coxsackie B myocarditis post pharyngitis

His prognosis is (multiple true-false)

a. Good because he is young.
b. Poor because of renal failure.
c. Good because he contracted his illness in an "epidemic" rather than "sporadic" form.
d. Poor because of fluid overload.
e. Good because he sought medical care promptly.
f. Poor because he did not seek medical care promptly.

3. A 49 year old mildly obese alcoholic white male executive presented to the ER with L flank pain radiating to the groin which was intermittent, colicky, and severe. Two years earlier he had been seen in the same ER for an acutely swollen, hot, painful R great toe but did not seek ongoing care after emergency treatment.

You should consider ordering (multiple true-false):

a. KUB
b. UA
c. CXR
d. Foot X-ray
e. IVP
f. BE

His most probable metabolic problem deals with (choose one):

a. Calcium
b. Glucose
c. Alcohol
d. Lipids
e. Uric acid

Treatment includes (multiple true-false):

a. Dietary modification
b. High fluid intake
c. High fiber intake
d. Thiazide diuretic
e. Colchicine
f. Nonsteroidals
g. Allopurinol
h. Aspirin

4. The number one cause of hyponatremia in hospitalized patients is

a. syndrome of inappropriate antidiuretic hormone (SIADH)
b. congestive heart failure
c. dehydration
d. infusion of hypotonic solutions

5. Laboratory values showing a BUN of 50, a creatinine of 6, a urinary sodium of 60, a urine osmolality of 200, and a urine sediment showing renal epithelial cells is more indicative of

a. acute tubular acidosis
b. prerenal azotemia

6. The cause(s) of papillary necrosis of the kidneys include (multiple true-false)

a. analgesic abuse
b. diabetes
c. sickle cell anemia
d. pyelonephritis
e. polycystic kidney

7. Struvite renal stones (comprised of magnesium, ammonia and phosphate) are caused by urea-splitting bacteria and give a characteristic

   a. low urine pH
   b. high urine pH

XII. ANSWERS

1. b

   c

   a-True; b-True; c-True; d-False; e-True; f-False; g-False

2. c

   d

   a-True; b-False; c-True; d-False; e-False; f-False

3. a-True; b-True; c-False; d-False; e-True; f-False

   e

   a-True; b-True; c-False; d-False; e-False; f-False; g-True; h-False

4. a

5. a

6. a-True; b-True; c-True; d-True; e-False

7. b

CHAPTER 4: RHEUMATOLOGY - IMMUNOLOGY

I. **RHEUMATOID ARTHRITIS**

   A. Symptoms

   Bilaterally symmetrical inflamed small joints of hands
   (classic): MCP's, PIP's (DIP's are involved more
   in osteoarthritis); morning stiffness, lassitude.

   B. Signs

   Early: Red, hot swollen joints, low grade fever,
   elevated sedimentation rate, positive RA titer (may
   take several months)

   Late: ulnar deviation, rheumatoid nodules over
   extensor surfaces, subluxations, swan neck deformi-
   ties, pericarditis.

   C. Treatment

   1. NSAID's

   2. Physical therapy

   3. Plaquenil

   4. Gold

   5. Steroids (low dose po and intraarticular)

   6. Disease modifying agents: Methotrexate

   7. Synovectomy, joint replacement

II. SYSTEMIC LUPUS ERYTHEMATOSUS

A. Must have four or more of the following:

malar rash   discoid rash
arthritis (2 or more joints)   photosensitivity
hematologic disorder   oral ulcers
  hemolysis   proteinuria or
  leukopenia < 4000   cellular casts
  lymphopenia <1500   seizures or psychosis
  thrombocytopenia <100,000   immunologic disorder
serositis   false + VDRL,
  pleurisy or effusion   ANA, anti DNA,
  pericarditis   anti Sm
  peritonitis   + LE Prep

B. More common in blacks, orientals, some American Indians, females, may be familial

C. Disease of autoantibodies leading to inflammation and tissue injury. Lupus "band test" shows deposition of immunoglobulin and complement at the dermal-epidermal junction in clinically normal skin.

D.

Autoantibody	Disease
ANA	Lupus, MCTD, scleroderma many disorders with low titers
Anti native DNA	Lupus
Anti single stranded DNA	Lupus, drug induced lupus
Anti histone H2A-H2B	Drug induced lupus
Anti Smith	Lupus
Anti RNP (ribonuclear protein)	Lupus but high in mixed connective tissue disease (MCTD)
SS-A SS-B	Sjogren's

E. Drug Induced Lupus

1. Prototype is with procainamide, also seen with INH, phenytoin, griseofulvin, hydralazine

2. Get many of above criteria but do not get renal disease

3. Onset weeks to months after drug is begun, usually resolves with cessation of drug

4. Distinguish by history and above antibodies

   5. Positive ANA's occur in many patients on these
      drugs. That, <u>without symptoms</u>, does not consti-
      tute the syndrome and does not require drug
      cessation.

F. Lupus and Pregnancy

   1. High rate of miscarriage and stillbirth

   2. Postpartum flare of lupus may occur

   3. Infants may have thrombocytopenia and heart block
      due to transplacental passage of autoantibodies.

G. Treatment

   1. NSAID's for arthritis.

   2. Steroids, Plaquenil, 6-Mercaptopurine, plasma-
      pheresis (experimental) used for renal, CNS
      disease

III. <u>DEGENERATIVE JOINT DISEASE</u>

A. Symptoms

   1. Chronic pain and stiffness of knees, low back,
      hips, hands, cervical spine.

   2. Obesity and age are risk factors. "Wear and tear"
      arthritis.

B. Signs

   1. Minimal inflammation. May have tenderness,
      decreased range of motion.

   2. X-ray shows osteophytes, decreased joint space.

C. Treatment

   1. NSAID's, intraarticular steroids.

2. Physical therapy, joint replacement.

IV. **GOUT, PSEUDOGOUT**

A. Symptoms

1. Inflamed painful joint, usually monoarticular, classic podagra of great toe in gout

2. May occur post-op, or at bedrest.

B. Signs

1. Erythema, exquisite tenderness, swelling.

2. Crystals in neutrophils in joint fluid: uric acid in gout, calcium pyrophosphate in pseudo-gout.

C. Gout seen in obese alcoholic men on red meat diets. Rarely if ever in menstruating women.

V. **VASCULITIS**

Disease	At Risk	Primary Involved Organ	Pathology
Wegener's granulomatosis	Men	Respiratory tract and kidney	Necrotizing granulomata in small vessels
Goodpasture's	Men	Respiratory tract and kidney	Antiglomerular basement membrane antibody; HLA DRw2
Churg Strauss	Men	Lung	Allergic granulomatosis
Leukocytoclastic Vasculitis		Skin	Polymorphonuclear leukocytes in vessel wall
Hypersensitivity		Skin	Post drug reaction
Temporal arteritis	Elderly	CNS	Granulomata in artery
Lupus	Women	Kidney, skin	Anti DNA

Disease	At Risk	Primary Involved Organ	Pathology
Behcet's	Orientals, Mediterranean	Mouth and genital ulcers eye	Nonspecific
Thrombotic thrombocytopenia purpura	Young women	CNS, hemato-poietic, renal	Fibrin platelet clot in arteri-oles
Henoch-Schonlein purpura	Children, Young adults	Kidney, skin	Palpable purpura
Polyarteritis nodosa	Associated with Hepatitis B	Kidney, CNS	Aneurysms of medium arteries
Kawasaki	Children	Lymph nodes, coronary arteries	Aneurysms of coronary arteries

VI. SCLERODERMA

A. Systemic sclerosis is a generalized disorder of connective tissue.

    1. Symptoms

    a. Difficulty in opening mouth, swallowing; joint pain

    b. Raynaud's, dyspnea

    c. Diarrhea, esophageal reflux

    2. Signs

    a. Shiny atrophic "hide-bound" skin, poikilo-dermia (areas of hypopigmentation)

    b. Telangiectasias, Raynaud's, hypertension, renal failure

    3. Lab

    Positive ANA (Antinucleolar), Anti-Scl-70

4. Management

   Symptomatic Rx. Treat severe hypertension with ACE inhibitors, pericardial tamponade with window, acute pericarditis with steroids, overgrowth diarrhea with antibiotics, reflux with usual measures. At risk for lung cancer due to pulmonary fibrosis. Penicillamine has been used.

B. Localized Scleroderma (CREST)

   1. Calcinosis, calcified subcutaneous deposits, Raynaud's, esophageal motility disorder, sclero-dactyly, telangiectasia

   2. More limited disease, slower progression.

   3. Lab

      Anti-centromere antibody

VII. POLYMYOSITIS - DERMATOMYOSITIS

A. Symptoms

   1. Proximal muscle pain and stiffness

   2. Rash

B. Signs

   1. Tender muscles.

   2. Heliotrope (purplish) discoloration around eyes

   3. Gottron's sign (pathognomonic), erythematous papules over dosal interphalangeal joints

C. Lab

   1. Increased CPK and other muscle enzymes

   2. Abnormal EMG

   3. Abnormal muscle biopsy

   4. AntiJo/antibody (increased especially in subset with pulmonary fibrosis)

D. Dermatomyositis associated with malignancy of lung, colon, ovary, stomach, breast.

VIII. EOSINOPHILIA - MYALGIA SYNDROME

A. Observed after ingestion of tryptophan. Symptoms of diffuse muscle ache, fatigue.

B. Presence of leukocytosis, high sedimentation rate, eosinophilia.

C. Treat with prednisone.

D. May be fatal.

IX. POLYMYALGIA RHEUMATICA

A. Patients > 50 yrs, sed rate > 50.

B. Aching of shoulder and pelvic girdle muscles.

C. May have mild anemia.

D. Treat with low dose Prednisone (5 - 10 mg/day) with excellent response.

E. Symptoms similar to temporal arteritis.

X. TEMPORAL (GRANULOMATOUS) ARTERITIS (see above)

A. Also, patients complain of jaw claudication, visual loss, headache.

B. Consideration of the diagnosis and prompt institution of high dose steroids may be vision-saving.

C. Confirm diagnosis with temporal artery biopsy showing granulomas.

Disease	Serology/Lab	Site of Involvement	Treatment
Lupus	Anti DNA	Joints, muscle, kidney	NSAID's, steroids
RA	RA titer	Joints	NSAID's, MTX

Disease	Serology/Lab	Site of Involvement	Treatment
MCTD	Anti RNP		
Polymyositis	High CPK	Proximal muscles	Prednisone
Scleroderma	Antinucleolar Ab, Anti-Scl-70	Skin, smooth muscle	None satisfactory
Polymyalgia rheumatica	High sed rate	Shoulder and pelvic girdle	Low dose prednisone
Adult Still's (great question for FUO)	High WBC	Rash (transient during fever), splenomegaly, few joints	Aspirin
Cryoglobulinemia	Abnormal gamma globulins	Palpable purpura lower legs; kidney	Steroids, cytotoxic drugs, plasmapheresis
Sjogren's	Rheumatoid factor HLA-B8, DR3 or DR4, SS-A, SS-B	Eyes, salivary glands	Artificial tears and saliva, steroids

XI. LOW BACK PAIN

A. Disk Disease

    1. May have sudden onset of low back pain

    2. Pain may radiate down one leg, with or without numbness, with or without precipitating event.

B. Compression Fractures

    1. Thoracic vertebrae may collapse asymptomatically.

    2. Causes loss of height and "dowager's hump" in elderly women.

C. Osteoporosis

   1. Risk factors: female, fair, thin, smoking, alcohol, theophylline.

   2. Hip fracture common cause of morbidity and mortality in elderly women.

   3. Prevented by estrogen at menopause, exercise.

D. Degenerative Joint Disease

   1. Commonly associated with compression of vertebrae.

   2. Chronic pain. Common in cervical and lumbosacral. Rare in thoracic spine.

   3. Hypertrophic spurs, osteophytes on x-ray.

E. Facet Syndrome

   1. Pain with walking, improves with rest (pseudoclaudication).

   2. Diagnose with CT scan.

F. Muscle Spasm

   1. Common in herniated nucleus pulposus or torn annulus.

   2. Visible, palpable paravertebral spasm.

G. Spondyloarthropathy

   1. Ankylosing spondylitis: - X-ray "bamboo spine." Begins prior to age 30. Begins in sacroiliac joints (hot on bone scan) and moves cephalad. HLA-B27+.

   2. Reiter's syndrome - Associated urethritis, conjunctivitis, arthritis. HLA-B27+.

   3. Noninflammatory

      Spondylitis
      Spondylolisthesis

H. Cancer

Myeloma causes lytic lesions (classic: pt with low
back pain, high sed rate, anemia). Prostate
causes blastic lesions. Mnemonic for cancers
commonly metastasizing to bone "Pb Ktl" = lead kettle:

P - prostate (blastic)   K-kidney
B - breast   T-thyroid   (lytic)
    (blastic and lytic)   L-lung

I. Unusual causes (dissecting aneurysm, retroperitoneal
adenopathy, etc.) Listen to description of pain.
Examine for findings to indicate other system
involvement such as pulses, nodes, DTR's, evidence
of diabetes, leukocytosis, fever.

XII. **QUESTIONS**

1. Erythema chronicum migrans, fever, chills, migratory
    polyarthritis, neurologic, and cardiac disease are
    all findings in

    a. Lyme disease
    b. gout
    c. septic arthritis
    d. pseudogout
    e. polyarteritis nodosa

2. Symmetric arthritis, morning stiffness, cervical
    spine involvement, and development of sicca syndrome
    is most compatible with

    a. rheumatoid arthritis
    b. SLE
    c. scleroderma
    d. degenerative joint disease
    e. polyarteritis nodosa

3. The seronegative spondyloarthropathies include all
    but

    a. ankylosing spondylitis
    b. Reiter's syndrome
    c. psoriatic arthritis
    d. systemic lupus erythematosus
    e. inflammatory bowel disease

4. Drug-induced lupus is associated with

   a. hydralazine
   b. procainamide
   c. phenytoin
   d. isoniazid
   e. all of the above

5. Necrotizing vasculitis, granulomas of the upper and lower respiratory tracts, and glomerulonephritis are manifestations of

   a. Wegener's granulomatosis
   b. polyarteritis nodosa
   c. Henoch-Schonlein purpura
   d. erythema nodosum
   e. all of the above

6. An elderly patient has shoulder girdle stiffness and hip pain. His sedimentation rate is 85. The most likely diagnosis is (one best answer)

   a. rheumatoid arthritis
   b. lupus
   c. polymyalgia rheumatica
   d. polymyositis
   e. degenerative joint disease

7. Scleroderma has all of the following features EXCEPT

   a. telangiectasias
   b. diarrhea
   c. renal failure
   d. hypertension
   e. diabetes

8. Mortality from lupus is due to all but one of the following

   a. renal failure
   b. respiratory failure
   c. Libman-Sacks endocarditis

9. The diagnosis of lupus is made by a positive ANA.

   _____ True   _____ False

10. Arthrocentesis is important in the evaluation of monoarticular arthritis primarily to rule out (choose one)

    a. rheumatoid arthritis
    b. lupus
    c. vasculitis
    d. septic joint
    e. trauma

11. Temporal arteritis can be a medical emergency if untreated due to irreversible

    a. renal failure
    b. blindness
    c. muscle weakness
    d. respiratory failure
    e. cardiomyopathy

12. Chylous effusions contain

    a. uric acid crystals
    b. calcium pyrophosphate
    c. cholesterol
    d. porphyrins

13. Hepatitis B is associated with some cases of

    a. polymyositis
    b. polymyalgia rheumatica
    c. polyarteritis nodosa
    d. Caplan's syndrome
    e. lymphangioleiomyomatosis

14. The renal effects of nonsteroidals are most pro-nounced in which population?

    a. young women
    b. young men
    c. elderly women
    d. elderly men
    e. children

15. The gastrointestinal side effects of nonsteroidals can be minimized by which one of the following?

 a. administration with food
 b. use of antacids
 c. use of H2 blockers
 d. use of sucralfate
 e. use of misoprostel
 f. all of the above

16. Which bleeding diathesis(es) is/are associated with chronic polyarthritis? (multiple true-false)

 a. Von Willebrand's
 b. Coumadin use
 c. factor 8 deficiency
 d. factor 9 deficiency
 e. factor 13 deficiency
 f. autoimmune thrombocytopenia

17. Hazards of arthrocentesis include all EXCEPT

 a. sudden lowering of joint fluid pressure
 b. introduction of bacteria into joint space
 c. injecting corticosteroid into an infected joint
 d. needle stick injury to doctor
 e. corticosteroid induced pain flare

18. Gotryen's sign is pathognomonic of

 a. rheumatoid arthritis
 b. ankylosing spondylitis
 c. systemic lupus erythematosus
 d. discoid lupus
 e. dermatomyositis

19. Immunoglobulin staining of the dermal-epidermal junction in clinically normal skin is diagnostic of

 a. rheumatoid arthritis
 b. ankylosing spondylitis
 c. systemic lupus erythematosus
 d. discoid lupus
 e. dermatomyositis

20. All of the following are characteristic of ankylosing spondylitis EXCEPT

   a. low back pain begins before age 30
   b. HLA-B27 antigen present > 90%
   c. 30° oblique views of sacroiliac joints are helpful in showing sacroiliitis
   d. predominantly female sex
   e. "bamboo spine" decreases range of motion

XIII. **ANSWERS**

   1. a

   2. a

   3. d

   4. e

   5. a

   6. c

   7. e

   8. c

   9. False

   10. d

   11. b

   12. c

   13. c

14. d

15. f

16. a-False; b-False; c-True; d-True; e-False; f-False

17. a

18. e

19. c

20. d

CHAPTER 5: INFECTIOUS DISEASES

I. ACQUIRED IMMUNODEFICIENCY SYNDROME (AIDS)

This field is changing daily. Please refer to journal articles for updated information.

A. Acquisition of Virus

    1. Through shared body secretions: by sex, shared needles, blood transfusion.

    2. Increasing heterosexual transmission; infected prostitutes spreading the virus heterosexually is a major problem in third world countries.

    3. Seroconversion may be asymptomatic.

    4. Acute illness - Mono like illness: fatigue, fever, adenopathy, hepatosplenomegaly. May occur 6 weeks to 6 months.

B. CDC Proposed 1992 AIDS Surveillance and Case Definition for Adults and Adolescents.

Revision was proposed to simplify the existing system of numerous AIDS defining clinical diagnoses and to utilize the very important parameter of CD4 counts, upon which prognosis and therapy are based. It is included here because it makes sense.

Proposed Clinical Category

	A	B	C
	Asymptomatic, generalized lymphadenopathy, or primary HIV acute illness.	Symptomatic Not A or C (see below)	AIDS indicator condition (see below)
CD4 Category			
1. > 500/mm^3	A1	B1	C1
2. 200-499/mm^3	A2	B2	C2
3. < 200/mm^3 AIDS indicator cell count	A3	B3	C3

Proposed Category A (adolescent or adult)

1. asymptomatic HIV infection

2. persistent generalized lymphadenopathy

3. acute primary HIV illness or history thereof

4. no history of category B or C conditions

Proposed Category B conditions

1. attributed to HIV infection or cell mediated immune defect

2. include but not limited to

    * Bacterial endocarditis, meningitis, pneumonia or sepsis.

    * Candidiasis, vulvovaginal; persistent (> 1 month duration), or poorly responsive to therapy.

    * Candidiasis, oropharyngeal (thrush)

    * Cervical dysplasia, severe; or carcinoma

    * Constitutional symptoms, such as fever (> 38.5 degrees C) or diarrhea lasting > 1 month

* Hairy leukoplakia, oral

* Herpes zoster (shingles), involving at least two distinct episodes or more than one dermatome

* Idiopathic thrombocytopenic purpura

* Listeriosis

* Mycobacterium tuberculosis, pulmonary

* Nocardiosis

* Pelvic inflammatory disease

* Peripheral neuropathy

Proposed Category C conditions

1. Conditions listed in the 1987 surveillance case definition for AIDS in adolescents or adults.

2. Are strongly associated with severe immunodeficiency, occur frequently in HIV-infected individuals, and cause serious morbidity or mortality.

   List of conditions in the 1987 AIDS surveillance case definition:

   * Candidiasis of bronchi, trachea, or lungs

   * Candidiasis, esophageal

   * Coccidioidomycosis, disseminated or extrapulmonary

   * Cryptococcosis, extrapulmonary

   * Cryptosporidiosis, chronic intestinal (> 1 month duration)

   * Cytomegalovirus disease (other than liver, spleen, or nodes)

   * Cytomegalovirus retinitis (with loss of vision)

   * HIV encephalopathy

* Herpes simplex: chronic ulcer(s) (> 1 month duration): or bronchitis, pneumonitis, or esophagitis

* Histoplasmosis, disseminated or extrapulmonary

* Isosporiasis, chronic intestinal (> 1 month duration)

* Kaposi's sarcoma

* Lymphoma, Burkitt's (or equivalent term)

* Lymphoma, immunoblastic (or equivalent term)

* Lymphoma, primary in brain

* Mycobacterium avium complex or M. kansasii, disseminated or extrapulmonary

* Mycobacterium tuberculosis, disseminated or extrapulmonary

* Mycobacterium, other species or unidentified species, disseminated or extrapulmonary

* Pneumocystis carinii pneumonia

* Progressive multifocal leukoencephalopathy

* Salmonella septicemia, recurrent

* Toxoplasmosis of brain

* Wasting syndrome due to HIV

C. Associated Malignancy - Kaposi sarcoma (more common in gay men than other risk groups), lymphoma. Non-Hodgkins lymphoma has been linked to Epstein-Barr virus.

D. Ethical issues of underground drugs, scarce resources, termination or withholding of life support. Experimental drugs are being released by FDA unusually quickly.

E. General Therapeutic Recommendations 1992

1. Treat with antiretroviral drug therapy when CD4 < 500/mm^3.

Start with AZT, switch or add other (DDI or DDC), when progression occurs.

2. Prophylax for Pneumocystis when CD4 < 200/mm^3.

3. Use Hepatitis B, Pneumavax, influenza vaccines.

4. Treat associated infections: commonly multiple drugs for MAI, chronic diflucan for cryptococcal meningitis. Note: Mycobacterium tuberculosis is on the rise in US, partly due to AIDS, homelessness, injection drug use. Because of its virulence, TB occurs earlier in the natural history of HIV disease than the atypicals. Resistant TB is on the rise.

F. General Trends 1992

1. Less Pneumocystis being seen as the AIDS-indicating condition with advent of prophylaxis.

2. More Mycobacterium tuberculosis, particularly extrapulmonary.

3. More infected women with resultant maternal trans-mission to infants.

4. More heterosexual transmission.

II. LEGIONNAIRES' DISEASE

A. Symptoms

1. Dry cough and lack of other URI symptoms.

2. High fever, pleurisy, abdominal pain, prostration, confusion, watery diarrhea

B. Signs

1. Tachypnea and fever with a relatively slow pulse

2. Early rales, multilobe pneumonia, neurologic signs

3. Culture for usual organisms negative

4. Often SIADH

5. Anti-legionella serology shows a rise in titer between acute and convalescent serums.

6. High sed rate, elevated liver functions, hematuria, azotemia.

7. 15-20% mortality.

8. Radiographic resolution may take many weeks.

C. There are many species of Legionella, an aerobic weakly staining gram negative rod which must be cultured on media supplemented by cysteine, iron and charcoal. Spread by airborne route with a propensity for growth in water which then becomes aerosolized. Ex: cooling towers, humidifiers, industrial machinery.

D. Disease Occurs In Two Patterns

1. Pneumonia with a low attack rate of disease per person exposed and days' long incubation period.

2. Pontiac fever which has a high attack rate and hours' long incubation period. Clinically there is fever, headache, myalgia, malaise.

E. Treatment

1. Erythromycin, tetracycline, respiratory support.

2. No specific therapy needed for Pontiac fever.

III. **MYCOPLASMA INFECTIONS**

A. The Organism

1. Not a bacterium, not a virus

2. Size of large virus; smallest free living form

3. No cell wall, won't respond to penicillins

4. Cultures look like fried-egg

5. Pathogenicity

a. Prefers respiratory epithelium of host

b. Produces hydrogen peroxide which damages epithelium and red cell membranes leading to autoimmune hemolysis.

6. Remains in sputum even after appropriate antibiotics up to 30-40 days

7. Long incubation period of 2-3 weeks

8. Very common cause (up to 75%) of pneumonia in
   confined populations; a disease of young people

B. Symptoms

1. Fever, prominent cough (nonproductive), headache,
   burning chest pains.

2. Gradual onset as opposed to pneumococcus or
   influenza

C. Signs

1. Bullous myringitis in 15%, pleural effusion
   (small) in 15%, few rales.

2. Patient does not look sick. CXR looks worse than
   patient with extensive infiltrates in bilateral
   lower lobes. Has been called "walking pneumonia".

D. Autoimmune Manifestations

1. Cold agglutinins

   a. Hemolysis

   b. Raynaud's, acral gangrene (especially in
      sickle cell disease)

   c. Cerebrovascular accident when titer very high
      (thousands)

2. Stevens-Johnson syndrome (blistering skin and
   mucus membrane lesions)

3. False positive VDRL

E. Diagnosis

1. Proper clinical setting

2. Culture organism

3. Cold agglutinin > 1:32

4. Specific rising antibody titers

5. Ask about exposure to birds (R/O chlamydia)

F. Treatment

1. Erythromycin or tetracycline for two weeks.

IV. **TOXIC SHOCK SYNDROME**

Fever, rash, confusion, hypotension, diarrhea, liver function abnormalities, renal failure.

A. Menstrual

B. Nonmenstrual

Post operative wound infections; secondary to skin infections.

C. Non Staphylococcal

May have identical syndrome due to streptococcal toxin.

V. **URINARY TRACT INFECTIONS**

A. Acute Pyelonephritis

1. Symptoms and signs

a. Fever, flank pain

b. Pyuria, WBC casts, leukocytosis

c. May have abdominal pain, associated cystitis.

2. Pathogenesis

a. Look for obstruction: ureteral reflux, stone, bladder outlet secondary to BPH.

b. Associated diabetes, pregnancy.

3. Treatment - IV antibiotics

B. Cystitis

1. Symptoms of burning, frequency.

2. Hematuria.

C. Urosepsis

   1. Common in elderly nursing home patient.

   2. Prior dehydration, may have underlying urinary obstruction (stone, BPH).

VI. GUT ASSOCIATED INFECTIONS

A. Ludwig's Angina

Infection of floor of mouth. Mixed aerobic/anaerobic flora.

B. Boerhaave Esophagus

Ruptured esophagus with pain, left pleural effusion, mediastinitis, subcutaneous emphysema.

C. Acute Cholecystitis

RUQ pain and tenderness on palpation (positive Murphy's sign), fever, increased alkaline phosphatase, leukocytosis.

D. Ascending Cholangitis

Fever, jaundice, RUQ pain. Seen in patients with altered duct anatomy such as obstruction from tumor or surgery.

E. Typhlitis

Infection of colonic wall with gut flora seen in neutropenic patients. Requires surgical excision.

F. Diverticulitis

LLQ pain, fever, leukocytosis, possible palpable LLQ mass or fullness. Prevent with high fiber diets.

G. Perirectal Abscess

Painful defection, palpable induration, fever; seen in neutropenic patients.

VII. **TICK-BORNE INFECTIONS**

    A. Rocky Mountain Spotted Fever

        1. Rash classically involves palms and soles.

        2. Conjunctivitis, increased LFT's, DIC, seen during warm months.

        3. Need high index of suspicion. Tick bite may be inapparent.

    B. Lyme Disease (Borrelia burgdoferi)

        1. First sign is "erythema chronicum migrans"

        2. Neurologic signs such as Bell's palsy (CN VII) and meningitis

        3. Arthritis.

        4. Tick is very small.

        5. Treatment of skin lesions is with oral tetracycline, penicillin, or erythromycin for 10-20 days. Patients may worsen during first hours of therapy.

        6. Meningitis, cranial and peripheral neuropathy are treated with intravenous penicillin G, 20 million units daily for 10 days.

        7. Lyme arthritis is also treated with parenteral penicillin, IM benzathine penicillin 2.4 million units weekly for three weeks.

VIII. **PNEUMONIA (PROTOTYPE PNEUMOCOCCAL)**

This is so important you should read the section in a medicine textbook.

    A. Symptoms

        1. Sudden severe rigor, cough, rusty sputum.

        2. Fever, pleurisy, referred pain to shoulder or abdomen, dyspnea, malaise.

B. Physical Findings

1. Rales, signs of consolidation, (increased fremitus, E to A changes, bronchial breath sounds), splinting, rub.

2. Chest wall tenderness, respiratory distress, hypotension, shock.

C. Streptococcus pneumonia

1. Facultative anaerobe, occurs in pairs, gram positive.

2. Contains a polysaccharide capsule that promotes virulence (inhibits phagocytosis).

3. Is carried by healthy people who develop a viral upper respiratory infection followed by aspiration of and invasion by pneumococcus.

4. Pathophysiology (four stages)

a. Spreading wave of edema fluid containing pneumococci.

Spreads to anatomic barrier such as lobar fissure.

b. Older zone of consolidation with hemorrhage and immunologically recruited inflammatory cells in alveoli causing gross "red hepatization" of lung.

c. Oldest zone of resolution with predominantly leukocytes causing gross "gray hepatization" of lung.

d. The process heals usually without scarring. Macrophages clean up debris and are expectorated out by patient.

5. Diagnosis

a. Sputum gram stain. Look for many polys and few epithelial cells to know it's a good specimen.

b. Look for gram positive diplococci and the absence of other pathogens such as staph (gram positive clusters of cocci).

c.   Sputum culture

d.   Blood culture positive in 15-25% and confirms diagnosis.

e.   Counterimmunoelectrophoresis of urine and blood detects polysaccharide antigen and may be helpful if cultures are negative (most useful in meningitis on CSF).

f.   Type 3 pneumococcus very virulent and can cause rapidly fatal illness. Asplenic patients are particularly susceptible to pneumococcus as they lack ability to opsonize.

g.   Resistant organisms: 2-5% of isolates are penicillin resistant at an intermediate level.

h.   Treatment

1.   Outpatient with mild symptoms: oral penicillin or erythromycin X 7 d.

2.   Uncomplicated pneumonia: penicillin G, 1 million u IV every 6 hours X 7 d or procaine penicillin 600,000 u IM every 12 hours X 7 d.

3.   With meningitis, endocarditis, arthritis: High dose penicillin G, 3-4 million u IV every four hours X 10 d (meningitis), to 2-4 weeks (endocarditis).

D.

Bug	CXR Pattern	Sputum	Risk Factor
Streptococcus pneumonia	Lobar or segmental, RML	Rusty due to bleeding into alveoli	Asplenia, alcoholic, myeloma, hypogamma-globinemia, sickle cell disease, heart failure
Klebsiella	Cavity upper lobes, bulging interlobar fissure	Orange (blood and pus) or red currant jelly	Alcoholic

Bug	CXR Pattern	Sputum	Risk Factor
Hemophilus influenza type B	May resemble pneumococcus		Children < 5 years
Legionella	Bilateral patchy multilobe progress to lobar, segmental. May cavitate	Scant	Community acquired exposure to water vapor
Aspiration (mixed)	Right middle lobe/lower lobe		Decreased consciousness, tube feedings, impaired swallowing
Staphylococcus	Multiple patchy infiltrates that coalesce to pneumatoceles or abscesses		Nosocomial, post influenza, injection drug user

E. Vaccination

Candidates for Pneumovax

asplenic patients	diabetes
myeloma patients	over 65
COPD, asthma	sickle cell disease
heart disease	lymphoma, leukemia

IX. INFLUENZA

A. The virus

1. Influenza A is a different genus than Influenza B.

2. Antigenic variation: Surface glycoproteins possess hemagglutinins(H) or neuraminidases (N) and are important in identifying strains.

   a. Antigenic drift: A relatively minor change occurring frequently every few years. The strain is named by the year and site of the isolation.

      b. Antigenic <u>shift</u> is a major change that results from genetic reassortment of two different strains simultaneously infecting a single cell. A new hemagglutinin or new neuraminidase results; since there is no pre-existing immunity, a major outbreak occurs.

      c. Antigenic variation is responsible for epidemics and pandemics of disease.

3. Hemagglutinins are more important than neurinidases in the above antigenic variation and in the production of protective antibody.

4. The viruses present at the end of the flu season are the ones likely to begin the next season (herald wave phenomenon).

B. The Disease

1. Is transmitted person to person via respiratory secretions.

2. Has a short incubation period of 18-72 hours.

3. Causes respiratory epithelial cell death, denudation of tracheo-bronchial tree and susceptibility to pneumonia by the host.

4. Occurs in winter months, in epidemics lasting 2-6 weeks.

C. The Symptoms and Signs

1. Sudden onset of myalgia, fever, headache, malaise out of proportion to mild upper respiratory symptoms of nasal stuffiness, discharge, sneezing, sore throat.

2. Prominent eye symptoms: burning, photophobia, pain on movement.

3. Tracheal burning, dry cough, fever.

4. Cervical adenopathy, few rhonchi or rales.

5. Cough and malaise may continue for several weeks.

D. Complications

   1. Primary influenza pneumonia

      a. Can occur in young healthy persons.

      b. Rheumatic heart disease and other preexisting cardiac conditions risk factors.

      c. Causes adult respiratory distress syndrome.

      d. High mortality.

   2. Secondary bacterial pneumonia

      a. Streptococcus pneumoniae, Staphylococcus aureus, Hemophilus influenzae.

   3. Guillain Barre Syndrome

      a. Seen occasionally after influenza though no definite causation established.

      b. Seen after <u>swine flu</u> (only) vaccine.

   4. Reye's syndrome

      a. In children and adolescents who use aspirin during influenza and varicella.

      b. Vomiting, lethargy and seizures begin as viral syndrome is improving.

      c. Elevated transaminases, hepatomegaly, hypoglycemia.

      d. Mortality is 10%.

X. <u>**ACUTE OSTEOMYELITIS**</u>

A. Symptoms

   1. Fever, pain

   2. History of trauma to bone, endocarditis, surgery, diabetes, (especially diabetic foot ulcers), alcoholism.

B. Signs

    1. Tenderness, erythema

    2. Draining sinus tract, radiographic signs of bone destruction and new bone formation, positive bone scan.

C. Organisms

    1. Staphylococcus aureus, coagulase positive, most common

    2. Staphylococcus epidermidis with prosthetic devices (including infected IV lines)

    3. Salmonella in sickle cell patients

    4. Pseudomonas in injection drug users and burn patients

    5. Mycobacterium tuberculosis (Pott's disease of spine)

    6. Anaerobes rare, usually in contiguity with anaerobic infections elsewhere

D. Management

    1. Obtain bone biopsy for culture if bug not isolated from blood

    2. Treat with appropriate IV antibiotics for an extended period (2-6 weeks), ascertain that blood levels of antibiotics are therapeutic (drug levels; Schlicter test)

    3. May require surgical debridement, sometimes repeatedly

    4. Diabetic foot ulcers contain multiple organisms and empiric therapy should cover Staph, E coli, anaerobes, Pseudomonas.

XI. <u>CNS INFECTIONS</u>

A. Encephalitis

    1. Usually viral, herpes I.

2. Fever, seizures, confusion should lead to lumbar puncture, EEG (temporal focus).

3. Empiric therapy with acyclovir has replaced brain biopsy due to the relative lack of toxicity of the former and the morbidity of the latter.

4. Herpes type I is the most common culprit in adult encephalitis. There is no correlation between presence of herpetic lesions in or around mouth and the presence of herpes in the brain.

5. Serologies with acute and chronic titers do not establish the diagnosis, and the virus can not be grown from CSF.

6. Have a high index of suspicion. Many patients present with behavioral abnormalities and are referred to a psychiatrist. When febrile, think of encephalitis.

B. Meningitis

1. Fever, headache, meningismus should lead to lumbar puncture.

2. History of otitis, head trauma with damaged cribriform plate (CSF rhinorrhea), basilar skull fracture, prior neurosurgery.

3. Meningococcal meningitis

a. A dramatic picture when full blown that all students should know.

b. History: often in the setting of confined groups (military recruits), acute onset of fever, headache, stiff neck, myalgia, rapidly progressing (over hours) to confusion, obtundation, stupor, coma, seizures.

c. Signs: Look for petechial, purpuric or ecchymotic rash. Signs of meningeal irritation (Kernig, Brudzinski's signs), but may be decreased or absent if deeply comatose. Hypotension, shock. Papilledema usually absent. Disseminated intravascular coagulation may be present.

d. Do urgent lumbar puncture followed by immediate high dose IV penicillin while fluid is going to laboratory.

e. Hemorrhagic adrenal infarction can be seen in this setting (Waterhouse-Friderichsen syndrome).

f. Meningococcemia can occur without meningitis (20%) with malaise, myalgias, fever, chills, arthralgias. It can progress rapidly as above or run a chronic course lasting days to weeks with intermittent febrile episodes.

g. Vaccine useful for serogroup C and A but B is the major serotype in U.S.

4. <u>Recurrent</u> meningococcal or gonococcal disease:

a. May be due to deficiency of terminal complement components, C8 and C9, which cause lysis of the bacterium.

b. This is a great board question.

5. Streptococcal meningitis:

a. Look for underlying focus: acute otitis media, sinusitis, pneumonia;

b. Look for predisposing conditions: sickle cell disease, asplenia, alcoholism

c. Most common cause for permanent neurologic defects (especially deafness) in children; neuro deficit in 10-20% of survivors

d. Cerebrospinal fluid findings:

1. Early polymorphonuclear cells up to 10,000 per cc. If > 50,000 think ruptured abscess

2. Hypoglycorrhachia with CSF glucose usually below 40 mg/dl or < 50% of blood glucose. Due to abnormal glucose transport.

3. Protein > 100 mg/dl. If grams, think subarachnoid block

       4. High lactic acid levels lead to hyper-ventilation

       5. Positive counterimmunoelectrophoresis with pneumococcus, hemophilus, meningococcus

   6. Aseptic meningitis

      a. Symptoms of headache, fever, malaise, stiff neck

      b. Signs of mild meningismus. Patients do not look toxic.

      c. LP rules out bacterial meningitis. CSF has few cells, usually lymphocytes (except if very early in course), mildly elevated protein, normal glucose

      d. No specific therapy needed.

C. Cerebritis

In patients with bacterial endocarditis; symptoms of confusion, fever.

D. Brain Abscess

In patients with bacterial endocarditis, congenital heart disease with right to left shunts.

E. Epidural Abscess

In patients with back surgery, diabetes, history of sepsis.

XI. **HERPES VIRUS INFECTIONS**

A. Cytomegalovirus

   1. Acquired post natally

      a. Hepatitis

      A cause of non A, non B hepatitis. Associated mononucleosis type illness with more fever and sweats, less adenopathy than Epstein Barr virus.

      b. Pancreatitis

    c. Retinitis

       A common problem in AIDS patients.

          Causes blindness.

          Requires life long IV therapy with foscarnet or ganciclovir.

    d. Pneumonitis

       A common problem in transplant recipients. CMV-negative blood is used for transfusion of immunosuppressed patients.

    e. Colitis

       Seen in AIDS patients with ulcerative lesions.

    f. In urine

       Urine is a good specimen source for culture.

    g. May be asymptomatic.

2. Acquired in utero

    a. 1% of all births.

    b. Transmitted by reactivation of latent maternal virus or primary maternal infection.

    c. Common cause of fetal growth retardation, intracerebral calcification, hepatospleno-megaly, thrombocytopenia with purpuric rash, hemolysis.

    d. Associated learning disabilities, hearing impairment, cognitive problems.

3. Diagnosis

    a. Culture of affected tissue.

    b. Seroconversion or significant serologic increase in titer.

    c. Use of monoclonal antibodies, DNA hybridiza-tion, and fluorescent antibody techniques.

B. Ebstein-Barr Virus (EBV)

1. Infectious mononucleosis

   a. Young people

   b. Fever, malaise, pharyngitis, adenopathy, hepatosplenomegaly, palatal petechiae, IgM heterophile.

   c. EB virus infection of B lymphocytes and persistently replicates after clinical infection is resolved (latent virus).

2. Chronic fatigue syndrome

   a. Need definite objective findings of organ involvement along with symptoms of fatigue, malaise, sore throat, fever.

   b. Need definite antibody titers to EBV-specific antigens.

3. Lymphoma

   a. Burkitt type in Africa. Associated high titers to EBV.

   b. B cell in immunosuppressed patients (AIDS). EBV genome in tumor cells.

4. Nasopharyngeal cancer in China

   a. Patients have high antibody titers.

   b. Viral genome found in tumor cells.

C. Herpes Type 1 (in Adults)

1. See section on encephalitis.

2. Common cause of recurrent blisters at vermilion border, around mouth and nose. Exacerbations during stress, immunosuppression.

3. Herpetic whitlow of finger. Inoculation from active lesion. May be Herpes 2 with genital lesions primary source.

4. Along with type 2 can cause serious disease in AIDS patients with non-healing ulcers of skin, perirectal area.

5. Responds to lower doses of acyclovir than zoster. Can prevent recurrence with chronic therapy.

D. Herpes Zoster

1. Commonly occurs in Hodgkin's disease and lung cancer, especially after radiation therapy. May be seen with HIV.

2. Reactivation of varicella virus in dorsal root ganglion which causes eruption of vesicles in specific dermatome(s).

3. Pain and tingling may precede rash by days. When left anterior chest is involved can be mistaken for cardiac pain.

4. Can be treated with acyclovir 800 mg five times daily for 1 week.

5. Post herpetic neuralgia occurs commonly in the elderly (rare in the young); may require multimodal therapy with tricyclics, narcotics, nonsteroidals.

6. Motor involvement is very rare at 1%.

7. Trigeminal involvement with nasociliary extension to the eye can be predicted by vesicles at the tip of the nose and should prompt an ophthalmologic consult.

XII. ENDOCARDITIS

A. Symptoms

1. Fever, malaise, weakness.

2. History of dental work or invasive procedures, extensive dental caries, congenital heart disease, valvular heart disease, IV drug use, sepsis.

B. Physical Findings

    1. Embolic phenomena such as CVA, skin, splenic and renal infarcts; Roth spots in fundi, conjunctival petechiae.

    2. Splinter hemorrhages of nails; Osler's nodes of finger pads, Janeway lesions of palms and soles

    3. Heart murmur (changing)

C. Treatment

IV antibiotics in therapeutic doses for extended periods; surgery if above fails.

D. Prophylaxis

    1. At risk patients (see below)

    2. Normal patients, dirty procedure

    3. Normal patients, clean procedure but high morbidity if infection occurs

E. At Risk Patients

    1. Valvular heart disease

    2. Congenital heart disease

    3. Genitourinary procedures

    4. Open heart surgery

    5. Prosthetic device implantation

XIII. **QUESTIONS**

    1. In a known penicillin allergic patient, the incidence of allergy to a cephalosporin is approximately

        a. 10-15 percent
        b. 30 percent
        c. 50 percent
        d. 90 percent

2. The limiting factor in the use of Amphotericin B is its

   a. renal toxicity
   b. CNS toxicity
   c. phlebitis
   d. bone marrow suppression

3. Approximately two-thirds of episodes of septic shock are caused by gram-positive bacteria.

   _____ True   _____ False

4. The most common cause of infectious meningitis in the adult population is

   a. meningococcus
   b. pneumococcus
   c. *Haemophilus influenzae*
   d. listeriosis

5. A common cause of infectious meningitis in immunosuppressed patients is

   a. meningococcus
   b. pneumococcus
   c. *Haemophilus influenzae*
   d. listeriosis

6. A common cause of meningitis in military recruits is

   a. meningococcus
   b. pneumococcus
   c. *Haemophilus influenzae*
   d. listeriosis

7. A common cause of meningitis in alcoholics is

   a. meningococcus
   b. pneumococcus
   c. *Haemophilus influenzae*
   d. listeriosis

8. An organism most apt to cause pediatric meningitis is

    a. meningococcus
    b. pneumococcus
    c. *Haemophilus influenzae*
    d. listeriosis

9. Patients with a positive PPD and negative chest x-ray who are greater than 35 years of age are not treated with isoniazid because

    a. risk of hepatotoxicity is too great above this age
    b. too expensive
    c. outcome not altered
    d. there is no risk for recurrence

10. Roth's spots, Janeway lesions, embolic glomerulo-phritis, and Osler's nodes are all terms applied to

    a. drug fever
    b. infectious endocarditis (bacterial endocarditis)
    c. pneumococcal pneumonia
    d. myocarditis

11. Which of the following symptoms of urinary tract infections is most useful in pinpointing the source as being an upper versus a lower tract infection?

    a. dysuria
    b. frequency
    c. fever
    d. flank pain

12. The number one cause of cystitis in the outpatient population is

    a. *E. coli*
    b. pseudomonas
    c. serratia
    d. proteus

13. Brodie's abscess, sequestrum, and involucrum are terms used with

    a. osteomyelitis
    b. cellulitis
    c. erysipelas
    d. sepsis

14. A 20-year-old patient presents with fever, sore throat, enlarged tonsils, and bilateral posterior cervical adenopathy. The differential diagnosis includes all but one of the following

    a. streptococcal pharyngitis
    b. chlamydial pharyngitis
    c. infectious mononucleosis
    d. congenital rubella syndrome
    e. nasopharyngeal carcinoma
    f. cytomegalovirus

15. The causative organism in Lyme disease is

    a. Treponema pallidum
    b. Helicobacter
    c. Ixodides
    d. Borrelia burgdorferi
    e. Treponema (yaws)

16. A 50-year-old male oil executive presents with spiking fever and rigors. He has recently returned from a business trip to Kenya. To evaluate him, you do all of the following EXCEPT (choose one)

    a. ask about sexual intercourse with natives
    b. look at peripheral blood smear
    c. measure liver function tests
    d. palpate for splenomegaly
    e. check stools for ova and parasites
    f. order MRI of brain

17. River blindness may affect up to 40% of residents in Nigerian communities. It is due to (choose one)

    a. a tropical virus affecting the optic nerve
    b. onchocerciasis affecting skin and eyes
    c. echinococcal cyst in occipital lobe of brain
    d. tropical sprue leading to vitamin A deficiency
    e. oncogenic Epstein-Barr virus causing CNS lymphoma

18. The first step in dealing with a needlestick injury of a healthcare worker from a suspected hepatitis B patient is to (choose one)

    a. administer HBIG
    b. determine seropositivity of patient and seronegativity of healthcare worker
    c. administer hepatitis vaccine
    d. measure SGOT levels of patient
    e. administer interferon to healthcare worker

19. Actinomycosis causes human disease primarily (choose one)

    a. as an allergic response to fungus
    b. as a disseminated blood borne pathogen
    c. as an infection of the head and neck and chest
    d. as an abdominal mass
    e. as a cellulitis of the lower extremity

20. The 1992 OSHA (Occupational Safety Health Administration) rules prohibit (choose one)

    a. double gloving for HIV patients
    b. hand washing after degloving
    c. recapping of needles
    d. safety goggles for potential splashes
    e. mandatory HIV testing of healthcare workers

21. Rocky Mountain Spotted Fever resembles measles (rubeola) clinically EXCEPT for (choose one)

    a. fever
    b. conjunctivitis
    c. rash
    d. Koplick spot
    e. age

22. The parvovirus of Fifth disease also causes (choose one)

    a. sickle cell anemia
    b. leukemia
    c. aplastic anemia
    d. lymphoma
    e. disseminated intravascular coagulation

23. Risk factors for lower extremity erysipelas include all but (choose one)

    a. diabetes
    b. lung cancer
    c. obesity
    d. venous stasis
    e. athlete's foot

24. One of the following unique advantages of the quinoline antibiotic is (choose one)

    a. its oral effectiveness against pseudomonas
    b. its usefulness in COPD
    c. its usefulness in UTI
    d. its interaction with theophylline
    e. its cost

25. The acquisition of HIV is facilitated by all EXCEPT (choose one)

    a. coexistent herpes
    b. coexistent syphilis
    c. anal intercourse
    d. condom use

26. Toxoplasmosis of the brain in AIDS patients is often confused with

    a. lymphoma
    b. cryptococcal meningitis
    c. HIV dementia
    d. vincristine neuropathy
    e. cerebral atrophy

27. A 25-year-old black male hospitalized on the psychiatric floor develops high fever and confusion. CBC shows leukocytosis. You want to consider all EXCEPT

    a. pneumococcal sepsis due to underlying sickle cell disease
    b. salmonella sepsis due to underlying HIV disease
    c. salmonella sepsis due to underlying sickle cell disease
    d. neuroleptic malignant syndrome from antipsychotic medication
    e. clozapine induced WBC dyscrasia

28. Infections requiring intact healthy macrophages for containment include all but one

    a. mycobacterium tuberculosis
    b. brucellosis
    c. tularemia
    d. HIV

29. Malaria and sickle cell anemia are endemic in the same parts of Africa because

    a. both genomes are transmitted by the same species of mosquito
    b. treatment of malaria is more efficacious in sickle cell patients, leading to a survival advantage
    c. sickled red cells are resistant to malarial infection
    d. sickle cell patients are frequently hospitalized, protecting them from the bite of the mosquito

30. A 29-year-old black male presents with odynophagia (painful swallowing). You notice a 20 pound weight loss in his chart and a history of anorectal disease. He denies homosexual activity. Physical exam reveals oral thrush. His underlying disease is (choose one)

    a. peptic acid induced stricture
    b. herpes esophagitis
    c. candida esophagitis
    d. AIDS/HIV
    e. esophageal carcinoma

31. Allergic rhinitis may be <u>distinguished</u> from the common cold by (multiple true-false)

    a. improvement with decongestants
    b. presence of sneezing and coughing
    c. presence of clear nasal discharge
    d. presence of eosinophilia
    e. presence of pale swollen nasal mucosa
    f. occurrence during spring and fall

32. Entameba histolytic causes (multiple true-false)

    a. colitis
    b. flask shaped ulcers on biopsy
    c. eosinophil tissue infiltration
    d. toxic megacolon
    e. disease in travelers
    f. disease which may be confirmed serologically

33. Simultaneous jaundice and renal failure are seen in (multiple true-false)

    a. leptospirosis
    b. Rocky Mountain Spotted Fever
    c. carbon tetrachloride poisoning
    d. carbon monoxide poisoning
    e. thrombotic thrombocytopenia purpura

34. Diarrheal syndromes with resulting arthralgia/ arthritis include (multiple true-false)

    a. yersinia
    b. intestinal bypass for obesity
    c. campylobacter jejuni
    d. quinidine diarrhea
    e. inflammatory bowel disease
    f. salmonella

35. Chagas disease causes "sleeping sickness" and cardio-myopathy. The responsible agent is a(n) (choose one)

    a. neurotropic virus
    b. mycobacterium
    c. HTLV-1 found in the Caribbean
    d. trympanosome
    e. fluke

36. Schistosomiasis haematobium is a fluke which causes (multiple true-false)

    a. hematuria
    b. bladder cancer
    c. decreased bladder contractility and capacity
    d. bladder fistulae to gut
    e. painful micturition

37. Physicians caring for patients returning from the 1992 Barcelona Olympics were warned of (choose one)

    a. toxic oil syndrome originating in Spain
    b. liver disease resulting from steroid use in athletes
    c. rhabdomyolysis in runners
    d. penicillin resistant pneumococci
    e. Legionnaire's disease from water vapors

38. Grouped vesicles should bring to mind (multiple true-false)

    a. herpes zoster
    b. herpes simplex
    c. pityriasis rosea
    d. herpetic whitlow
    e. drug reaction

XIV. **ANSWERS**

    1. a

    2. a

    3. True

    4. b

    5. d

    6. a

7. b

8. c

9. a

10. b

11. c

12. a

13. a

14. d

15. d

16. f

17. b

18. b

19. c

20. c

21. d

22. c

23. b

24. a

25. d

26. a

27. e

28. d

29. c

30. d

31. a-False; b-False; c-False; d-True; e-True; f-False

32. a-True; b-True; c-True; d-True; e-True; f-True

33. a-True; b-True; c-True; d-False; e-True

34. a-True; b-True; c-True; d-False; e-True; f-True

35. d

36. a-True; b-True; c-True; d-True; e-True

37. d

38. a-True; b-True; c-False; d-True; e-False

CHAPTER 6: GASTROENTEROLOGY

I. ORAL

A. Ulcers

   1. Aphthous: In chemotherapy, connective tissue diseases, stress.

   2. Herpetic: Grouped vesicles in or around mouth and nose, anterior to Stenson's (parotid) duct in mouth (posterior are usually Coxsackie B).

   3. Fungal: Especially infectious in histoplasmosis (common bug in Oklahoma and Midwest).

B. Periodontal Disease

   1. Risk factor for aspiration, sepsis, endocarditis, lung abscess, brain abscess

C. Cancers

   1. Risk factors: alcohol, tobacco

   2. All mucosa at risk in aerodigestive tract with these risk factors. Second cancers common, and Vitamin A may help prevent.

II. ESOPHAGUS

A. Motility Disorders

   1. Achalasia

   2. Gastroesophageal reflux disease (GERD) - Very common symptom. Patient may complain of chest pain or acid taste, common after eating, on

reclining, in obesity, pregnancy, with tight garments, bending over. Worse with calcium blockers, chocolate, alcohol.

3. Spasm - May resemble angina pectoris and may be relieved by nitroglycerin.

4. Stricture - Patient complains of difficulty swallowing (dysphagia) or painful swallowing (odynophagia); sequela of severe reflux or radiation therapy. May need mechanical dilation.

5. Webbing - Associated with iron deficiency; "Plummer-Vinson" disease in females.

B. Barrett's esophagus - Metaplasia secondary to acid disease, at risk for malignant transformation.

C. Cancer

1. Squamous of mid esophagus

2. Adenocarcinoma of gastroesophageal junction

3. Risk factors: alcohol, tobacco.

4. High mortality (95 + %) despite therapy.

D. Bleeding

1. Variceal secondary to portal hypertension - treated with sclerosis, propranolol to decrease portal pressure.

2. Ulceration

3. Mallory-Weiss tear - Common with vomiting; usually resolves rapidly.

E. Rupture - Boerhaave's - Patient may complain of heartburn, dysphagia, odynophagia.

F. Infections - May need biopsy with culture to distinguish. Seen in compromised host.

1. Candida - Look for oral thrush; have a high index of suspicion in HIV patients and those undergoing radiation therapy.

2. Herpes

        3. CMV

III. <u>STOMACH</u>

A. Peptic Acid Disease

    1. Gastritis

    2. Duodenal ulcer - Recent role for Helicobacter pylori in pathogenesis of duodenal and gastric ulcer. Treat refractory patients with tetracycline, metronidazole, Pepto Bismol and H2 blockers.

B. Gastric Ulcer - see above

C. Nonsteroidals

Often use H2 blockers or sucralfate to protect stomach while using NSAID's. If refractory can use misoprostel.

D. Cancer

Declining incidence in this century. Increased with preservatives and smoked foods.

E. Surgeries

Marked decline since advent of H2 blockers. A number of now older patients underwent these surgeries and present with several syndromes. More on this later.

IV. <u>SMALL BOWEL</u>

A. Malabsorption States

    1. Terminal ileum disease

        a. lack of absorption of B12 and bile salts

        b. clinically presents with diarrhea, anemia

        c. visualize with small bowel barium x-ray or, if lucky, colonoscopy with extension into terminal ileum

        d. commonly due to Crohn's, gluten sensitive enteropathy (sprue), or terminal ileum resection

    e.   associated with renal stones due to hyperabsorption of oxalate by colon. This is an important concept. The stones which are formed are calcium oxalate and can actually be prevented by exogenous oral calcium to bind oxalate in the gut and prevent its absorption.

    f.   treat bile salt diarrhea with cholestyramine if < 100 cm of terminal ileum diseased or gone, B12 deficiency with injections

2. Fat malabsorption

    a.   foul-smelling stools with odor that lingers and causes complaints.

    b.   requires 72 hour stool collection for fat to document (not commonly done; may look for stool fat with Oil Red O stain).

    c.   associated lab features: prolonged protime due to decreased Vitamin K; decreased serum carotene.

    d.   may be due to pancreatic disease and not small bowel disease. May have history of pancreatitis, see calcifications in pancreas on KUB; treat with enzyme replacement.

3. Surgically constructed

    a.   jejuno-ilial bypass for obesity

        1.   associated with reactive arthritis, fatty liver

        2.   no longer performed

    b.   duodenal ulcer surgery

        1.   Billroth procedures with partial gastrectomy and bypass of proximal small bowel; not commonly done with advent of H2 blockers

        2.   associated long-term iron deficiency anemia due to need of acid and duodenum to absorb iron. This is a common clinical problem which may be refractory to oral iron.

3. occasional B12 deficiency due to lack of intrinsic factor if extensive gastrectomy. "Pernicious anemia" may be present without anemia. Screen patients with high MCV's.

B. Syndromes

1. Postoperative after ulcer surgery - Dumping syndrome: weakness, syncope, sweats, fatigue due to hyperinsulinemia/hypoglycemia and volume shifts from sudden load of carbohydrate.

2. Post small bowel resection - Short bowel syndrome if > 100 cm ileum resected. Diarrhea may respond to low fat diet.

C. Enteritis

1. Viral syndromes - "Gastroenteritis" with nausea, vomiting, diarrhea secondary to Norwalk agent, Rotavirus, enteroviruses.

2. Bacterial infections - Look for stool polys on smear in patients with fever, leukocytosis, diarrhea. Salmonella, Shigella, Yersinia, Campylobacter.

3. Post infectious arthropathy - Reactive after infections as in #2. HLA-B27 common.

4. Histoplasmosis in AIDS patients in Oklahoma - Abdominal pain, mass; usually found at surgery.

V. **COLON DISORDERS**

A. Motility

1. "Spastic" colon - More common in women. Patient needs to have structural pathology excluded.

a. unusually due to fiber lack

b. associated stress - Very important!

c. Treat with fiber, counseling, anti-spasmodics.

2. Laxative abuse

a. results in "sluggish" colon, melanosis coli

      b.   retrain bowel with fiber, stool softeners

    3. Prolonged transit times (rare) - Can document by swallow of radiopaque marker and daily KUB. More than 3 days is abnormal.

B. Redundant Colon

    1. Common in elderly

    2. Results in removal of water from stool throughout its long length causing hard stools, constipation and dehydration, can progress to serious illness and sepsis in elderly.

    3. Treat with fiber, stool softeners. If patient has above obtundation-dehydration syndrome, hospitalize, culture, fluids, antibiotics, supportive care.

C. Diverticulosis

    1. Usually in descending colon

    2. May bleed, usually stops spontaneously

    3. Requires fiber

D. Diverticulitis

    1. Left lower quadrant pain and fever

    2. Middle aged to elderly

    3. May heal with walled off abscess, fistula formation to bladder, vagina. These need surgical correction.

    4. May require surgical intervention for ruptured diverticulum/acute abdomen.

E. Angiodysplasia

    1. A common cause of lower GI bleeding; diagnosed at colonoscopy, rarely with tagged red cell studies, may be missed at autopsy.

    2. Associated in cecum and ascending colon with aortic stenosis in elderly. No reasonable reason for this but you should know the association.

3. Associated with smoking and increased platelet counts.

F. Colon Cancer

1. Second most common cancer in Americans (considering men and women together)

2. Genetic influence:

   a. Hereditary polyp syndromes (Gardner's and familial polyposis) which degenerate to cancer by age 40

   b. Hereditary tendency to polyps

   c. Cancer-prone families

3. High dietary fat increases incidence. Know this.

4. Polyps have increased malignant potential with increased size: > 3 cm, 30% malignant. Polyp formation decreased with sulindac.

5. Screen with stool hemoccults, rectal exams, flexible sigmoidoscopy (controversial regarding cost-effectiveness of screening). Screen persons in #2, and persons over 50 years when incidence rises.

6. Must explain positive stool hemoccult or iron deficiency; requires GI work up. Common question: patient > 50 years, asymptomatic and microcytic red cells. You need to R/O cecal cancer.

7. Effective postoperative adjuvant chemotherapy with 5FU and levamisole for patients with lymph node involvement (Dukes' Stage C) to prevent recurrence.

G. Rectal Cancer

1. Same risk factors as colon cancer. Must explain rectal bleeding; don't assume secondary to hemorrhoids without work-up.

2. Undiagnosed or untreated, leads to painful neural plexus involvement.

3. Effective postoperative adjuvant therapy with 5FU and radiation for patients beyond Stage A (mucosal disease only) to prevent recurrence

H. Inflammatory Bowel Disease

1. Ulcerative colitis

   a. Limited to colon mucosa (rectum always involved) and "backwash ileitis" into terminal ileum

   b. Radiographic findings: loss of haustral markings, "collar button ulcers". Barium should not be given to acutely ill patient.

   c. Gut manifestations cured with colectomy

   d. Extra-intestinal manifestations of arthritis, spondylitis, fatty liver, pericholangitis, sclerosing cholangitis, chronic active hepatitis, cirrhosis, pyoderma gangrenosum of skin.

   e. Risk of cancer increases with pancolitis and length of disease greater than ten years, dysplasia on biopsy.

   f. Treat with 5ASA, Azulfidine, corticosteroids, colectomy, now have continence preserving surgery

   g. Toxic megacolon is a grave complication with fever, abdominal pain, distention and tenderness, absent bowel sounds, and dilated mid-transverse colon to 6 cm on plain film. May be precipitated by antidiarrheal medications, narcotics, anticholinergics, hypokalemia, bowel prep, barium enema.

2. Crohn's disease

   a. Entire thickness of bowel wall involved, may have skip areas (normal segments adjacent to diseased segments) which grossly are called "pseudopolyps".

   b. May involve small bowel, colon (anywhere along GI tract)

   c. Radiography: cobblestone appearance due to alternation of ulcers and normal mucosa, segmental narrowing, "string sign"

   d. Tendency to fistula formation

    e. Surgery does not cure; can recur in remaining bowel.

    f. Treat with corticosteroids, bowel rest with parenteral hyperalimentation

    g. Extra-intestinal manifestations similar to ulcerative colitis.

I. Anal Disease

1. Fistula

Common in Crohn's, tuberculosis

2. Hemorrhoids

    a. bleeding

Possible to become iron deficient and very anemic (e.g. Hgb = 4 g)

    b. thrombosed

        1. painful

        2. may be incised and removed

        3. office banding techniques

    c. bulk fiber laxatives important

3. Perirectal abscess or inflammation common in leukemics, AIDS

4. Proctitis

    a. common in gay men; post-radiation for prostate cancer or rectal cancer; inflammatory bowel disease

    b. treat specifically with antibiotics if infectious

    c. treat inflammation with cortisone enemas if noninfectious

VI. <u>GALLBLADDER</u>

A. Acute Cholecystitis

1. May have few symptoms in elderly. May be precipitated by weight loss, CABG, lipid lowering drugs. Common in 4F's: fat, female, fecund, forty.

B. Chronic Cholelithiasis

1. Medical management with drugs (ursodeoxycholic acid) to solubilize stones; requires ongoing therapy; expensive.

2. Surgical management; laparoscopic cholecystectomy useful in high risk patients.

VII. <u>PANCREAS</u>

A. Pancreatitis

1. Acute: Abdominal (epigastric) pain radiating to back. Nausea and vomiting.

a. Causes of pancreatitis

Alcohol (very common)	Drugs
Gallstones (acute,	DDI
not chronic)	Hydrochlorothiazide
Hypertriglyceridemia	Sulfa
Lupus	L asparaginase
Viral	
Mumps, CMV	

b. Management: NPO, occasionally NG tube, hydration, pain medication, H2 blockers usually used. Antibiotics don't help. Get alcohol rehab, treat any underlying condition.

c. Complications:

Hemorrhagic pancreatitis - develop shock, Grey-Turner sign (flank ecchymosis); get surgeons to see.

Pseudocyst - develop mass seen on ultrasound, may resolve or require marsupialization by surgery.

Hypocalcemia - Calcium may precipitate out with fat: saponification.

Fat necrosis - Weber Christian syndrome.

Acute tubular necrosis from dehydration, shock

Adult respiratory distress syndrome

2. Chronic

   a. May develop recurrent acute pancreatitis even in absence of continued alcohol.

   b. May develop pancreatic calcifications on x-ray ("chronic pancreatitis"), pancreatic insufficiency, diabetes if > 90% function lost.

B. Carcinoma

   1. Head of pancreas

      a. Symptoms: weight loss, abdominal pain; jaundice is _early_ due to common duct obstruction. Dyspepsia.

      b. Signs: painless jaundice, with palpable gallbladder: "Courvoisier's gallbladder"

      c. management - even "early" surgery does not cure.

   2. Tail of pancreas

      a. Symptoms: weight loss, usually dramatic, back and abdominal pain. Jaundice is _late_ due to liver metastases.

      b. Signs: none early enough to help. Late ascites, hepatomegaly, jaundice, increased alkaline phosphatase and GGTP.

      c. Management: usually only palliation with pain control, psychological support of patient and family.

VIII. <u>LIVER</u>

A. Hepatocellular Disease

1. Viral hepatitis - usually SGPT higher than SGOT. Reversed in alcoholic liver disease.

a. Hepatitis

1. A small RNA virus transmitted by fecal-oral route.

2. Short incubation period of 2-6 weeks.

3. Common in day care centers.

4. Associated with prodrome of urticaria (yellow hives), pruritis, loss of taste for cigarettes, monoarticular arthritis. Many anicteric cases.

5. Diagnose with anti Hep A (IgM).

6. Resolves without chronic disease.

7. May rarely get fulminant hepatic necrosis and aplastic anemia but less often than in other forms of viral hepatitis.

b. Hepatitis B

1. Worldwide significance: responsible for much morbidity and mortality, causes hepatoma, #1 cancer in world

2. DNA virus, transmitted by shared body secretions, long incubation period (1-6 months, average 50 days)

3. Serology:

Acutely get rise in "Dane particle" markers; e antigen (HB e Ag), viral DNA (HBV DNA), DNA polymerase (DNA p, transient)

Next get rise in liver enzymes, surface antigen (HB s Ag), and core antibody (anti-HBc). The latter is a sensitive marker of hepatitis B infection, present (IgM) or past (IgG). A negative test for anti-HBc excludes the diagnosis.

Next get rise in surface antibody (anti-HBs) which is made 5-6 months after acquisition of virus. It is _protective_. (If found early in the work-up of hepatitis, it likely reflects _remote_ hepatitis B and excludes Hepatitis B as the cause of the present problem). This is the point where the patient should be clinically improving with normalizing liver functions. If not, consider liver biopsy to exclude chronic active hepatitis.

Chronic carrier state occurs in 10% of patients with hepatitis B.

4. Extra-hepatic manifestations more common than in hepatitis A with rashes, glomerulonephritis, arthritis due to immune complexes. Think about hepatitis B in polyarteritis nodosa, where 30% are surface antigen positive.

5. Vaccine available from recombinant technology in yeast. Induces surface antibody (anti-HBs). Should be given to at-risk populations.

6. At-risk populations:

   Health care professionals in contact with blood and body fluid

   Homosexuals

   Injection drug users

   Down's syndrome

   Dialysis patients

   Babies of infected mothers

7. Vertical transmission:

   Mother to offspring, especially likely if mother develops acute Hepatitis B in late pregnancy or early post partum, has Hepatitis B e Ag, or has chronic hepatitis. Important in developing countries.

8. Use of Hepatitis B immune globulin (HBIG):

   In cases of parenteral exposure of seronegative recipient to seropositive donor

   Use in conjunction with vaccine

c. Hepatitis D (delta agent):

   1. An incomplete RNA virus which requires presence of Hepatitis B to infect host cell

   2. Exists in plasma, coated by Hepatitis B surface antigen

   3. Found in injection drug users

   4. In patients chronically infected with hepatitis B, infection with D can cause either chronic active hepatitis or fulminant hepatic failure.

d. Hepatitis C and non-A, non-B:

   1. Serologies difficult (C) or non-existent

   2. Common cause for transfusion-related hepatitis, since screening has occurred for hepatitis B since 1972.

2. Toxins

Necrosis	Increased transaminases	Cholestasis	Granuloma	Fibrosis	Neoplasia (adenoma & carcinoma)	Fatty Liver	Hepatic vein thrombosis	Peliosis hepatis
Acetaminophen (dose dependent)	Aspirin (juvenile RA)	Chlorpromazine (systemic symptoms)	Halothane	Methotrexate	Estrogens	Tetracycline	6 thioguanine	Estrogens
		Erythromycin estolate (fever, RUQ pain)	Phenytoin	6 mercapto-purine	Androgens	Valproic acid		Androgens
	Methyldopa (chronic active hepatitis)	Estrogens (pruritis)	Allopurinol		Danazol	Alcohol		
	Rifampin (induces P-450)		Quinidine			Aspirin in Reye's syndrome		
	INH (age > 35)							

    a. Chemical - carbon tetrachloride, vinyl chloride, thorium dioxide (old radioisotope used in scans).

    b. Biological - aflatoxin, liver flukes, echinococcal cysts, ameba.

3. Inflammatory diseases

    a. Chronic active hepatitis - diagnose by liver biopsy.

    If due to Hepatitis B, can treat with interferon. May have anti smooth muscle antibody, usually not in conjunction with hepatitis B.

    b. Chronic persistent hepatitis - usually "triaditis" on biopsy, no treatment required.

4. Inherited diseases

    a. Alpha-1-antitrypsin deficiency:

       1. Macronodular cirrhosis

       2. Suspect with abnormal serum protein electrophoresis in proper clinical setting.

       3. Associated emphysema

    b. Wilson's disease

       1. Homozygous recessive in young people

       2. May present as recurrent acute _hepatitis_, cirrhosis

       3. May present with _neurologic_ or psychiatric symptoms: dystonia, dysarthria, tremor

       4. Defect in copper excretion into bile. Copper stored in liver, then redistributes causing _Kayser-Fleischer_ rings in cornea; _hemolytic anemia_ and _neurologic_ change

       5. Decreased serum ceruloplasmin in 95%, increased hepatic copper on biopsy > 250 mg/g dry weight

        6.   Treat with penicillamine to prevent death from cirrhosis

   c.   Hemochromatosis

        1.   Common (1/200 to 1/600) genetic disorder of increased iron absorption and deposition into organ <u>parenchyma</u>. (This causes damage; storage in reticuloendothelial cells as in hemosiderosis is more benign)

        2.   HLA linked to A3, increased B7 and B14.

        3.   Sex prevalence same but clinical disease more often male 10:1 due to factors such as blood loss through menstruation and pregnancy, alcohol intake, food intake.

        4.   Bronze skin (melanin and hemosiderin), arthritis, diabetes, hypogonadism, cardiomyopathy, cirrhosis, hepatoma.

B.   Biliary Tract Disease

   1.   Stones

      a.   Gallbladder

         1.   Probably need treatment.

         2.   Newer forms of therapy include laparascopic cholecystectomy (risk of damage to common duct, vascular structures) and drug to dissolve stones (expensive and must be given chronically).

      b.   Common duct

         1.   Stones need to be attended to.

         2.   This structure is easily scarred by inflammation and surgery and can create chronic problems.

         3.   Secondary biliary cirrhosis can develop with chronic common duct obstruction.

   2.   Drugs

      a.   Granulomatous hepatitis (see prior table)

    b.   Obstructive patterns - (increased alkaline phosphatase, increased GGTP)

3.   Inflammatory diseases

    a.   Sclerosing cholangitis

        1.   Associated with inflammatory bowel disease

        2.   Chronic narrowing of bile ducts intervening with normal areas, leading to characteristic <u>beaded</u> appearance on cholangiography.

    b.   Primary biliary cirrhosis - seen in middle-aged women. Associated itching, hypercholesterolemia, antimitochondrial antibody. Great question for exams.

C. Fibrosing Diseases

1.   Cirrhosis

    a.   Alcoholic (micronodular)

    b.   Macronodular secondary to viral hepatitis, alpha-1-antitrypsin deficiency.

2.   Fibrosis secondary to drugs - Methotrexate, 6 mercaptopurine

D. Blood Vessel Disease

1.   Portal hypertension

    a.   Results from increase in pressure in portal vein or tributaries due to increase in portal venous blood flow (rare) or increased resistance to venous flow (common).

    b.   Manifest clinically as variceal bleeding, ascites, portal-systemic collaterals, splenomegaly.

2.   Diseases causing portal hypertension

    a.   Diseases of liver.

        1.   Cirrhosis (all causes): Regenerating liver nodules and bands of fibrosis compress and

  narrow vessels with distortion and reduction in the sinusoidal bed.

  2. Infiltrative diseases: (infectious as Schistosomiasis, chronic inflammatory as sarcoidosis).

  3. Alcoholic hepatitis

 b. Diseases of vessels/heart

  1. Thrombosis of portal vein

  2. Thrombosis of hepatic veins

  3. Veno occlusive disease

  4. Congestive heart failure

 c. Diseases of increased blood flow

  1. Splenomegaly

  2. Arteriovenous fistulae

3. Vasculitis

E. Liver Failure

1. Fluids and electrolytes

 a. Hyponatremia, hypokalemia, low BUN

 b. Fluid retention, hyperaldosteronism, metabolic alkalosis

 c. Treat with salt and fluid restriction, bed rest, Aldactone

 d. Diuresis can be dangerous and precipitate hepatorenal syndrome.

2. Encephalopathy

 a. Precipitated by GI bleed, sepsis, protein load.

 b. Associated asterixis (liver flap).

 c. Manage with lactulose, neomycin, protein restriction.

3. Bleeding

    a. May be due to varices or commonly, peptic ulcer.

    b. Varices can be sclerosed; decrease portal pressure with propranolol.

4. Hepatorenal Syndrome

    a. Occurs in advanced liver disease, usually alcoholic cirrhosis.

    b. Occurs after sudden fluid shifts such as vigorous diuresis, GI bleed, or paracentesis.

    c. The kidneys act as if pre-renal azotemia existed with very low urine flow and low urine sodium. The process is irreversible and fatal. The patient dies however, *in* renal failure rather than *of* renal failure. The kidneys can be transplanted to a patient with a normal liver and they work well.

F. Primary Peritonitis

1. Seen in cirrhotics with ascites.

2. Patient develops fever, leukocytosis and abdominal pain and tenderness.

3. Diagnose with paracentesis, examine fluid for leukocytes, bacteria and culture.

4. Treat for gram negatives.

5. High mortality rate.

G. Hepatoma

1. Relation to Hepatitis B - most common cancer worldwide due to prevalence of Hepatitis B infection.

2. Relation to alcohol - underlying cirrhosis almost always present.

3. Symptoms - weight loss, pain, dyspepsia; not early enough to make a difference in survival. Screening at-risk population with alpha fetoprotein does not diagnose early enough for cure.

4. Signs - ascites, palpable mass, bruit over liver due to vascularity, increased LFT's, increased alpha fetoprotein.

IX. THE EFFECTS OF ALCOHOL AND SMOKING ON THE GI TRACT

A. Aerodigestive Tract Cancer

1. Oropharyngeal, tongue, nasopharyngeal

2. Esophageal

B. Esophagus

1. Esophagitis, Mallory-Weiss tear, varices

C. Stomach

1. Gastritis

2. Peptic ulcer disease

D. Liver

1. Fatty liver

a. May be asymptomatic or mildly symptomatic with tender hepatomegaly.

b. Not specific for alcohol: fat seen with steroids, diabetes, jejunal bypass for obesity.

c. Reversible with discontinuation of alcohol.

d. Excellent prognosis.

2. Alcoholic hepatitis

a. Triad of fever, hepatomegaly, leukocytosis.

b. Patients appear sick, bacterial infections must be excluded.

c. SGOT (AST) elevated (< 10 x normal) and higher than SGPT (ALT) which may be normal. Increased MCV.

d. Jaundice may be present.

e. Alcoholic hyaline not specific.

f. May progress to cirrhosis or to hepatic failure.

3. Cirrhosis

a. Related to average daily consumption of alcohol (4.5 oz., may be less for women) for 10-15 years, genetics, nutrition.

b. Asymptomatic in 10-20%.

c. May present with alcoholic hepatitis or complications of cirrhosis (ascites, variceal bleed, encephalopathy).

d. Labs as above. Bilirubin slightly increased, multifactorial anemia with folate deficiency, blood loss, hemolysis.

e. Better prognosis if no complications and abstinence from alcohol (60% 5 year survival).

X. QUESTIONS

1. The causes of upper GI bleeding include

   a. peptic ulcer disease
   b. esophageal varices
   c. Mallory-Weiss tears
   d. all of the above
   e. none of the above

2. Angiodysplasia of the large bowel is usually asymptomatic.

   _____ True   _____ False

3. The most common site of peptic ulcer disease is in the

   a. duodenum
   b. gastric fundus

4. The most probable etiology of diarrhea in a patient with significant bloating and abdominal pain who recently travelled to the mountains would be

   a. Giardiasis
   b. amoebic enteritis
   c. traveler's diarrhea
   d. Staphylococcal food poisoning

5. Malabsorption could be caused by

   a. bile salt deficiency
   b. pancreatic insufficiency
   c. mucosal abnormalities
   d. lactase deficiency
   e. all of the above

6. A colonic biopsy showing transmural inflammation, skip areas, noncaseating granulomas, and cobble-stoning on gross appearance would most likely represent

   a. ulcerative colitis
   b. Crohn's disease
   c. celiac sprue
   d. tropical sprue

7. Sclerosing cholangitis and pericholangitis are most associated with

   a. ulcerative colitis
   b. Crohn's disease
   c. celiac sprue
   d. tropical sprue

8. The most common causes of acute pancreatitis in the U.S.A. are biliary tract diseases and alcoholism.

   _____ True   _____ False

9. A 40-year-old white female presenting with jaundice, pruritis and laboratory abnormalities revealing a very high alkaline phosphatase, high cholesterol, high bilirubin, and a positive anti-mitochondrial antibody would most likely have

    a. primary biliary cirrhosis
    b. Wilson's disease
    c. hemochromatosis
    d. hepatoma

10. Precipitants of hepatic encephalopathy include

    a. sedatives
    b. an increased dietary protein load
    c. gastrointestinal bleeding
    d. diuretics
    e. all of the above

11. A 35-year-old white male presented to the ER with epigastric pain and vomiting. A blood specimen sent to the lab came back with "milky serum" noted on the report. His abdominal pain is likely due to

    a. peptic ulcer disease
    b. stomach cancer
    c. irritable bowel syndrome
    d. incarcerated inguinal hernia
    e. pancreatitis

12. The above patient has "milky serum" likely due to

    a. high HDL cholesterol
    b. high LDL cholesterol
    c. high triglycerides
    d. low LDL cholesterol
    e. recent ingestion of fatty meal

13. A common accompanying disease of the above situation is

    a. diabetes mellitus
    b. chronic calcific pancreatitis
    c. ulcerative colitis
    d. Crohn's disease
    e. hypothyroidism

14. A 56-year-old white male has been anticoagulated for recurrent deep venous thrombosis. While on Warfarin he experiences a GI bleed. Which of the following is/are true? (multiple true-false)

    a. The bleeding is due to Warfarin and need not be further explored.
    b. Anticoagulation may have unmasked a colon cancer or polyp.
    c. The patient may have an underlying protein deficiency.
    d. The patient may have a hypercoagulable state due to an occult carcinoma.
    e. The patient should have a total body CT scan.

15. The serum gastrin is high in which of the following disorders? (multiple true-false)

    a. pernicious anemia
    b. achlorhydria
    c. Zollinger Ellison syndrome
    d. gastric cancer
    e. gastrojejunostomy with retained antrum

16. A 70-year-old woman with congestive cardiomyopathy presents with crampy left abdominal pain, weight loss, and a positive stool hemoccult. "Thumb printing" distal to the splenic flexure is seen on x-ray. Her diagnosis is

    a. colorectal cancer
    b. diverticulitis
    c. inflammatory bowel disease
    d. volvulus of sigmoid
    e. ischemic colitis

17. A 27-year-old male presents with diarrhea, right lower gradient pain, and post prandial cramping of two months' duration. He has lost 10 pounds. Exam reveals a tender right lower quadrant and a positive stool hemoccult. His diagnosis is

    a. colorectal cancer
    b. diverticulitis
    c. inflammatory bowel disease
    d. volvulus of sigmoid
    e. ischemic colitis

18. A 64-year-old white male with a history of colon polyps presents with dull left lower quadrant pain and pain on sitting. He notes his stools have been difficult to pass and have been blood tinged. His diagnosis is

   a. colorectal cancer
   b. diverticulitis
   c. inflammatory bowel disease
   d. volvulus of sigmoid
   e. ischemic colitis

19. An 18-year-old girl presents with micrographia and slurred speech. A cousin had recently undergone a liver transplant. Her diagnosis is

   a. Early onset familial Parkinson's
   b. Toxoplasmosis
   c. Wilson disease
   d. Hansen disease
   e. Hodgkin disease

20. A 35-year-old white male alcoholic had abnormal liver functions presumed secondary to drinking. An astute medical student noted that he had grayish skin and abnormal glucose metabolism. His diagnosis is

   a. alcoholic hepatitis
   b. Wilson disease
   c. alcoholic pancreatitis
   d. sclerosing cholangitis
   e. hemochromatosis

21. Which of the following cause(s) pigment (calcium bilirubinate) gallstones? (multiple true-false)

   a. hereditary spherocytosis
   b. hereditary ovalocytosis
   c. sickle cell disease
   d. thalassemia major
   e. autoimmune Coombs' positive anemia

22. Risk factors to cause cholesterol gallstones include all but one of the following

    a. vagotomy and pyloroplasty
    b. female
    c. fecund
    d. middle age
    e. rapid weight loss
    f. carcinoma of gallbladder
    g. lipid lowering drugs

23. A young white woman with a known history of Graves' disease presents with hepatomegaly, spider angiomata, elevated liver functions, and arthralgias. She is likely to have

    a. alcoholic liver disease
    b. fatty liver of pregnancy
    c. lupoid hepatitis
    d. inflammatory bowel disease
    e. complication of radioiodine for Graves'

24. The characteristic laboratory abnormalities of primary biliary cirrhosis are

    a. elevated alkaline phosphatase, cholesterol, antimitochondrial antibody
    b. elevated alkaline phosphatase, cholesterol, smooth muscle antibody
    c. elevated serum carotene, protime, direct bilirubin
    d. elevated serum carotene, protime, indirect bilirubin
    e. elevated cholesterol, low albumin, elevated creatinine

25. Medical management of portal hypertension includes the use of

    a. captopril
    b. aspirin
    c. diltiazem
    d. nifedipine
    e. propranolol

26. Patients with known esophageal varices often bleed from other than their varices. A common (50%) site is from

   a. gastritis
   b. duodenal ulcer
   c. Mallory Weiss tear
   d. gastric polyps
   e. gastric cancer

XI. **ANSWERS**

   1. d

   2. True

   3. a

   4. a

   5. e

   6. b

   7. a

   8. True

   9. a

   10. e

   11. e

   12. c

   13. a

14. a-False; b-True; c-True; d-True; e-False

15. a-True; b-True; c-True; d-False; e-True

16. e

17. c

18. a

19. c

20. e

21. a-True; b-True; c-True; d-True; e-False

22. f

23. c

24. a

25. e

26. b

CHAPTER 7: OCULAR MANIFESTATIONS OF SYSTEMIC DISEASE

I. **DECREASED VISION**

A. Visual Field Cuts

1. Cerebrovascular accidents

2. Emboli to retinal arteries causing arterial thrombosis

3. Hypercoagulable states (high platelets, high proteins, high leukocytes) causing arteriolar and venous thrombosis

4. "Tunnel vision" secondary to pituitary adenomas

B. Monocular Visual Loss

1. Carotid artery embolization

2. Retinal detachment secondary to diabetic neovascularization and hemorrhage

3. Tumors, such as melanoma, optic nerve glioma

4. Lens displacement in Marfan's and homocystinuria

5. Optic neuritis in multiple sclerosis

6. Optic atrophy

C. Bilateral visual loss

1. With headache in temporal arteritis

2. With papilledema in brain tumors or intracerebral bleeds

      3. Chorioretinitis

          a. cytomegalovirus in AIDS

          b. histoplasmosis

      4. Uveitis

          a. sarcoidosis

          b. Reiter's syndrome

          c. Wegener's granulomatosis

II. THE RED EYE

A. Conjunctivitis

    1. Viral

        a. adenovirus

        b. measles

    2. Bacterial

    3. Chlamydial

    4. Drug-induced: 5 FU, Vitamin A

B. Keratitis

    1. Herpes simplex

    2. Herpes zoster as part of shingles of first division of trigeminal nerve

    3. Contact lens contaminants

C. Uveitis

    1. Systemic inflammatory disease (Sarcoid)

D. Glaucoma

Narrow angle may be precipitated by anticholinergic drugs used orally to treat systemic disease and by inhalation to treat COPD.

E. Seen with Graves' disease

Eye is proptotic with injected blood vessels.

F. Allergic

G. Orbital Cellulitis

H. Periorbital Cellulitis

III. **OTHER CAUSES OF ABNORMAL FUNDUS EXAM**

A. Blood Vessels

1. Hypertensive change

a. A-V nicking

b. hemorrhage

c. exudate

2. Diabetic change

a. microaneurysms

b. flame hemorrhage

c. exudate

1. soft cotton wool

2. hard waxy

d. neovasculization - requires laser therapy

3. Lupus change

a. cytoid body

4. Hyperlipidemia

a. color change to tomato soup or orange sherbet secondary to high triglycerides

5. Loss of venous pulsations in increased intra-cranial pressure

6. Subarachnoid hemorrhage causes subhyaloid retinal hemorrhage with a fluid level

B. Retinal Lesions

    1. Roth spots secondary to

        a. endocarditis

        b. systemic fungemia

        c. pernicious anemia

    2. Angioid streaks due to breaks in Bruch's membrane

        a. pseudoxanthoma elasticum

        b. sickle cell disease

    3. Retinal detachment

        a. traumatic

        b. spontaneous

    4. Tumors - ocular melanoma; has special propensity to metastasize to liver. Beware the patient with unilateral jaundice!

IV. DIPLOPIA

A. Cranial nerve palsy

    1. Diabetes

    2. Increased intracranial pressure

    3. Multiple sclerosis

B. Trapped or thickened extraocular muscles

    1. Graves' disease

    2. Blowout fracture

V. NYSTAGMUS

A. Dilantin toxicity

B. Multiple sclerosis

C. Brain stem lesions

D. Congenital

VI. PATIENT COMPLAINTS, NOT MUCH ON ROUTINE EXAM

A. Dry Eyes (sicca syndrome)

1. Sarcoidosis

2. Sjogren's syndrome

B. Blurred Vision

1. Diabetic swings in glucose causing osmotic change in lens

2. Error in refraction

3. Cataracts (early can be difficult to see with ophthalmoscope).

C. Pain

1. Glaucoma

2. Retrobulbar neuritis

3. Retrobulbar mass (lymphoma, infection)

VII. QUESTIONS

1. Sudden loss of vision in one eye, as the only symptom, is compatible with

    a. subdural hematoma
    b. seizure disorder
    c. cerebellar hemorrhage
    d. astrocytoma
    e. carotid embolization

2. The differential diagnosis of proptosis includes all but

    a. diabetic retinopathy
    b. Graves' ophthalmopathy
    c. retrobulbar lymphoma
    d. orbital cellulitis
    e. normal variant

3. Periorbital edema is associated with all of the following EXCEPT

   a. anasarca
   b. superior vena cava syndrome
   c. Addisonian crisis
   d. glomerulonephritis
   e. anaphylaxis
   f. congestive heart failure

4. The earliest retinal lesion in diabetics is

   a. waxy exudates
   b. cotton wool spots
   c. flame hemorrhages
   d. microaneurysms
   e. neovascularization

5. The diabetic retinal lesion requiring laser therapy
   is

   a. waxy exudates
   b. cotton wool spots
   c. flame hemorrhages
   d. microaneurysms
   e. neovascularization

6. A 40-year-old male patient presents to the emergency
   room having had a motor vehicle accident on the
   interstate highway. He stated that he never saw the
   car in the next lane. Visual field testing reveals
   tunnel vision. You should consider

   a. pituitary tumor
   b. pituitary apoplexy
   c. diabetic retinopathy
   d. cerebrovascular accident
   e. optic nerve glioma

7. A 35-year-old black female has a history of interstitial lung disease and lymphadenopathy showing non caseating granulomas on biopsy. She comes in now complaining of a red eye with visual loss. Her latest problem is

   a. viral conjunctivitis
   b. Graves' disease
   c. sarcoid uveitis
   d. tuberculous uveitis
   e. histoplasmosis

8. A 25-year-old immunocompromised white female is receiving total parenteral nutrition via a central line. She is spiking daily fevers though no septic focus has been found. From your daily fundoscopic exam, you astutely make the correct diagnosis of

   a. cytomegalovirus retinopathy
   b. diabetic retinopathy
   c. cholesterol embolization
   d. fungal sepsis from central line
   e. hypersensitivity to central line plastic

9. A 37-year-old HIV positive white male comes to you because of a painful facial rash involving one side of his forehead. You diagnose herpes zoster and consider immediate ophthalmologic referral if

   a. the rash involves the cheek below the eye implying involvement of more than the first trigeminal division
   b. the rash involves the tip of the nose implying nasociliary ganglion involvement
   c. the rash involves the entire body, implying dissemination
   d. the rash has spread across the midline making zoster less likely
   e. The rash is atypically hemorrhagic implying thrombocytopenia

10. A 29-year-old black female presents with double vision. Exam reveals a left sixth nerve palsy. The differential diagnosis includes all but one of the following

   a. diabetic neuropathy
   b. Graves' disease
   c. anorexia nervosa
   d. pseudotumor cerebri
   e. Lyme disease

11. Ptosis of the eyelid suggests

   a. third nerve involvement
   b. expanding aneurysm of internal carotid artery
   c. diabetic neuropathy
   d. myasthenia gravis
   e. all of the above

VIII. **ANSWERS**

1. e

2. a

3. c

4. d

5. e

6. a

7. c

8. d

9. b

10. c

11. e

CHAPTER 8: PSYCHOPHYSIOLOGIC SYNDROMES

These are very common clinical problems.

I. **MUSCULOSKELETAL**

   A. Fibrositis

      1. Upper back pain

      2. Shoulder and neck pain

      3. Trigger points

      4. Sleep disturbance

      5. Treat with reassurance, NSAID's, antidepressants, physical therapy.

   B. Chest Pain

      1. Intercostal muscle pain

      2. Costochondral pain

      3. Fear of cardiac disease

   C. Tension Headache

      1. Increased muscle tension of neck muscles

      2. Radiates from base of spine over to forehead

      3. Worsened by anxiety

      4. "Band-like" pain

D. Low Back Pain

    1. May be triggered by injury

    2. Secondary gain - worker's compensation and role of the "sick person" in the family

    3. Depression!

II. **CENTRAL NERVOUS SYSTEM**

A. Migraine Headache

    1. In genetically predisposed individuals; related to serotonin metabolism.

    2. Precipitated by emotions and other physiocochemical events, such as menses, alcohol, chocolate

B. Pseudoseizures

    1. Use of prolactin to differentiate - within 30 minutes of true seizure, prolactin level should be high.

    2. Secondary gain

C. Hyperventilation

    1. Tingling of fingers and circumoral area. This is physiologic. Try it yourself.

    2. May be associated with tachycardia, chest pain

D. Depression

    1. Magnifies "normal" aches and pains

    2. If one symptom treated, likely will develop a new one

    3. Tricyclics modify pain syndromes of depression

    4. Counseling an important adjunct

E. Anxiety

    1. Panic attacks

      a. sudden onset of "spells", fear of choking or not being able to breathe

      b. genetically linked, can be chemically reproduced

      c. need to be treated, as may develop into agoraphobia, then depression

      d. respond to benzodiazepines, tricyclics, MAO inhibitors

2. Generalized anxiety disorder

      a. six months or more duration to diagnose

      b. not situational

      c. heightened awareness, always "on alert"

      d. may need medication and psychotherapy

3. Obsessive compulsive behavior

      a. ritualized behavior

      b. responds to clomipramine

4. Fatigue

      a. rule-out hypothyroidism, anemia, hepatitis, viral syndromes

      b. consider depression

III. GASTROINTESTINAL

A. Irritable bowel syndrome

1. Alternating diarrhea and constipation

2. Gas

3. Pain in multiple abdominal sites

B. Organic states confused with irritable bowel

1. Lactose intolerance

2. Bezoars secondary to foreign body ingestion (hair, paper)

3. Short bowel syndrome

4. Partial small bowel obstruction

5. Narcotic bowel syndrome

6. Use of constipating medicines

7. High bulk diets

8. Ischemic bowel, vasculitis

9. Giardiasis

VI.   QUESTIONS

1.   A 35-year-old white female presents with complaints of headaches characterized by band-like pressure around the forehead and back of neck. They occur frequently and the patient takes aspirin, Tylenol, and Darvocet even in anticipation of the headache. The onset of the headaches correlated temporarily with marital separation. The best diagnosis is

   a.   migraine headache
   b.   cluster headache
   c.   chronic daily headache
   d.   stress
   e.   depression

2.   The best technique for managing this patient's headache is

   a.   counseling
   b.   addition of a nonsteroidal antiinflammatory
   c.   additional of a tricyclic
   d.   addition of a serotonin re-uptake inhibitor
   e.   withdrawal of all pain medication and institution of a tricyclic for prophylaxis

3. A 42-year-old white female executive complains of grouped ulcerations around the lip when under periods of stress at work. The most likely diagnosis is

   a. herpetic whitlow
   b. herpes zoster
   c. herpes simplex
   d. aphthous ulcers
   e. trigeminal neuralgia

4. A 57-year-old overweight hypertensive male smoker presents to the emergency room complaining of chest pain and a sense of impending doom. The latter symptom raises the likelihood of all but one of the following

   a. myocardial infarction
   b. pulmonary embolus
   c. dissecting aortic aneurysm
   d. cervical spine arthritis
   e. ventricular tachycardia, sustained

5. The diagnosis of irritable bowel syndrome requires all but one of the following

   a. biopsy proven colonic inflammation
   b. alternating diarrhea and constipation
   c. no structural bowel disease
   d. no lactase deficiency
   e. no parasitic infiltration

6. The following patients are at increased risk of sudden death EXCEPT

   a. a 65-year-old black male with diabetes and peripheral vascular disease
   b. an 83-year-old healthy white male whose wife of 60 years just died
   c. a 50-year-old hypertensive white male who just received word that he was passed over for a much wanted promotion
   d. a 37-year-old female who just gave birth
   e. a 42-year-old schizophrenic woman whose mother and aunt both died suddenly and unexpectedly at age 42

7. A young "up-and-coming" politician comes to you because of nervousness prior to speeches. This performance anxiety can be prevented with

   a. small doses of alcohol prior to speech
   b. small doses of propranolol prior to speech
   c. small doses of benzodiazepine prior to speech
   d. memorizing the speech
   e. practicing the speech

8. The key symptom of depression is

   a. anorexia
   b. early morning awakening
   c. multiple aches and pains
   d. crying spells
   e. anhedonia

9. The most stressful setting is

   a. feeling fatigued from too much work
   b. feeling lost in a new environment
   c. feeling powerless to change the environment
   d. feeling happy in a new relationship
   e. feeling sad at the end of a relationship

10. Alcoholics drink because

    a. alcohol makes them feel "normal" or good
    b. they are weak
    c. they have no self-discipline
    d. they have a well defined, established chemical abnormality
    e. they learned to do it to obtain secondary gain

11. The most successful treatment program for an alcoholic is

    a. Antabuse
    b. behavioral modification
    c. a 12 step alcoholic anonymous group
    d. combination therapy with clonidine and Librium
    e. psychoanalysis

VII. **ANSWERS**

1. c

2. e

3. c

4. d

5. a

6. d

7. b

8. e

9. c

10. a

11. c

CHAPTER 9:   HEMATOLOGY

Even practicing physicians can have a hard time remembering these
anemias, so we'll classify them in several ways and you can use
the one that makes the most sense to you.

I.   ANEMIAS, CLASSIFIED BY RBC SIZE

A.   Microcytic (small red cells)

Disease	RBC size (micra)	RBC Number	Fe	TIBC	Ferritin
Iron deficiency	55-80	<5 million	decreased	decreased	decreased (a <u>low</u> ferritin means iron lack)
Beta Thalassemia (trait)	60-78	>5 million	decreased	decreased	increased (confirm with hemoglobin electrophoresis)
Chronic disease	70's	<5 million	decreased	decreased	increased

B.   Macrocytic (large red cells)

Disease	RBC size	Retic Count	LDH	Risk Factors
Pernicious anemia	>100	<1%	very high (may be >1000)	s/p gastrectomy, elderly, other autoimmune (thyroid, adrenal) terminal ileum disease. Do not have to have anemia to have macrocytes and neurologic disease

Disease	RBC size	Retic Count	LDH	Risk Factors
Folate deficiency	>100	<1%	high	Alcoholism, pregnancy, hemolysis, starvation
Hemolysis	>100	high (may be 70% in enz def)	high	Drugs (Alphamethyldopa classic), autoimmune disease splenomegaly
Myelodysplasia	>100	<1%	normal	prior chemotherapy, abnormal chromosome, elderly

C. Normocytic

   Acute blood loss
   Chronic disease
   Hemolytic
   Aplastic
   Hemoglobinopathies
   Toxins
   Drugs

II. ANEMIAS, CLASSIFIED BY BONE MARROW MORPHOLOGY

A. Hypoplastic (Hypoproliferative)

Few red cell precursors on bone marrow aspirate or biopsy.

1. Etiologies

   Iron deficiency
   Chronic disease
   Aplastic anemia
   Injuries due to toxins: chemotherapy, insecticides, drugs

B. Hyperplastic (Hyperproliferative)

Many "spicules" seen grossly on aspirate at the bedside.

1. Definition: ineffective intramedullary (within the bone marrow) erythropoiesis

2. Etiologies:

    a. Vitamin deficiency

        1. B12

        2. Folate

    b. Hemoglobinopathies

        1. Sickle cell disease

        2. Hemoglobin C

    c. Genetic disorders with hemolysis

        1. Thalassemia syndromes

        2. Enzyme deficiencies (G-6-P-D)

        3. Hereditary spherocytosis

    d. Acquired disorders with hemolysis

        1. Drug induced (Alphamethyldopa)

        2. Paroxysmal nocturnal hemoglobinuria

        3. Autoimmune (lupus)

        4. Microangiopathic anemia (disseminated intravascular coagulation, thrombotic thrombocytopenic purpura)

    e. Myeloproliferative states (see later, Disorders of Leukocytosis)

C. <u>Dysplastic</u>

Myelodysplastic syndromes

1. Heterogeneous group of clonal disorders of pluripotent hematopoietic stem cells with frequent anemia, infections, bleeding, and evolution to acute leukemia.

    a. Hematopoiesis is ineffective.

    b. Global dysfunction of hematopoiesis with qualitative and quantitative abnormalities of RBC, neutrophils and platelets.

  c. Bone marrow necessary to assess degree of blasts (if overt acute leukemia, needs treatment).

2. Clinical features:

  a. Median age 68, equal sex ratio, median Hgb 9.0, median neutrophil count 1.7, median platelet count 108,000 median survival 10 months.

  b. Major symptoms: fatigue (89%), fever (24%), bleeding (24%), weight loss (29%), normal exam (28%), enlarged spleen (17%), enlarged liver (12%), petechiae/purpura (26%), progression to leukemia (27%)

  c. FAB subtypes

	Median survival/mo.
Refractory anemia	64
Refractory anemia with ring sideroblasts	71
Refractory anemia with excess blasts	7
Chronic myelomonocytic leukemia	8
Refractory anemia with excess blasts	8
Refractory anemia with excess blasts in transformation	5

  d. Treatment:

  Little value

   Pyridoxine, pyridoxalphosphate, androgens, steroids, low dose cytarabine, hydroxy-urea.

  Supportive care

   Transfuse
   Treat infections
   May need platelet transfusion if bleeding (even with adequate count) due to dysfunction.

Colony stimulating factors

> Erythropoietin (Epogen)
> Granulocyte CSF

Bone marrow transplantation if young

D. <u>Fibrotic</u>

Myelofibrosis

1. Extramedullary ("ectopic") hematopoiesis with marrow fibrosis and hypercellularity.

2. Clinical features

   Common over age 50, occasionally young women, progressive anemia, hepatosplenomegaly, fever, night sweats, weight loss; splenic infarction, portal hypertension, impaired platelet function.

3. Lab features

   a. Peripheral blood:

      Teardrop RBC's, immature myeloid cells, normoblasts ("leukoerythroblastic peripheral blood smear")

      Anemia, leukocytosis; platelets can be increased, normal, decreased.

   b. Bone marrow:

      Increased megakaryocytes
      Increased reticulin (fibrosis)
      Some patients have extensive osteosclerosis.
      Marrow fibroblasts are <u>not</u> involved with the abnormal clone.
      Myelofibrosis is <u>reactive</u> to the malignant pluripotent hematopoietic stem cell.

   c. Hyperuricemia, folate deficiency secondary to high cell turnover.

4. Natural history

   a. Conversion to acute leukemia < 10%, especially if alkylators used.

      b. Chronic illness, median survival 5 years, may go > 30 years.

    5. Treatment

      a. Splenectomy (does not improve survival) Reserved for well documented hypersplenism with severe cytopenia or major physical discomfort. Latter better treated with radiation or hydroxyurea.

      b. Supportive; transfuse

E. Myelophthisic (Bone Marrow Replacement States)

    1. Tumors

    2. Infections

    3. Granulomas

    4. Storage diseases (Gaucher's)

III. **DISEASES OF THE SPLEEN**

A. Role of the Spleen

Scavenger for the reticuloendothelial system; important for opsonization.

B. Hypersplenism

    1. Secondary to portal hypertension, common in cirrhotics

    2. Secondary to autoimmune diseases

      a. Lupus

      b. ITP (or ATP, autoimmune thrombocytopenia purpura). In this disease the spleen is active and hot on scan but not enlarged on physical exam.

      c. Rheumatoid arthritis with Felty's syndrome. Elderly men with high rheumatoid titers.

    3. Secondary to infectious diseases

      a. Viral (HIV, mono, CMV)

      b.   Bacterial (i.e., endocarditis)

      c.   Parasitic (Kala azar)

4. Secondary to hemolysis (work hypertrophy)

5. Secondary to storage/infiltrative diseases

      a.   Gaucher's

      b.   Sarcoid

      c.   Amyloid

      d.   Granulomatous

6. Primary

      a.   Lymphomas/sarcomas

      b.   Hodgkin's disease

C. <u>Hyposplenism</u>

1. Diagnosis: by Howell-Jolly bodies (RBC nuclear remnants normally culled out by spleen) which stain blue on peripheral smear.

2. These patients at risk for encapsulated-organism infections and need Pneumovax.

3. Anatomic (asplenia)

      a.   Congenital

      b.   Acquired

          1.   Immune

          2.   Traumatic

4. Functional

      a.   Sickle cell disease and variants due to splenic infarction

      b.   Multiple myeloma

      c.   AIDS

      d.   Lymphoma

IV. **DISORDERS OF LEUKOCYTES**

    A. Leukopenias

        1. Due to bone marrow failure (decreased production)

            a. Aplastic anemia

            b. Toxins

            c. Drugs

                1. captopril

                2. phenothiazines

                3. propylthiouracil

                4. chemotherapy

                5. many others

            d. Myelophthisic disorders

            e. Leukemias, lymphomas

            f. Infections

            g. Cyclic neutropenia

        2. Due to peripheral destruction

            a. Hypersplenism

            b. Felty's syndrome

    B. Leukocytosis (Quantitative Abnormality)

        1. Leukemoid reactions - high LAP score (stain for leukocyte alkaline phosphatase).

        2. Leukemia

            a. Chronic granulocytic - mature polys on smear, low LAP score, look for Philadelphia chromosome. (t9:22 translocation of C-abl proto-oncogene, just memorize it)

b. Acute granulocytic (there are several names for this entity, see below) blasts on smear, <u>Auer rods</u> in blasts, few mature polys, few platelets, anemia.

   1. Acute nonlymphocytic leukemia (probably preferred term)

   (acute granulocytic, acute myeloblastic, acute myelogenous)

      a. Diagnosis: > 30% blasts, peroxidase or sudan black positive

      b. FAB categories (7)

FAB	M1	myeloid without maturation
	M2	myeloid with maturation
	M3	promyelocytic (DIC) Associated DIC, may require heparin. Can be effectively treated with Vitamin A. Know this one.
	M4	myelomonocytic
	M5	monocytic - may get CNS involvement
	M6	erythroleukemia
	M7	megakaryocytic leukemia

   2. Cytogenetics: 50-60% of patients at diagnosis have abnormality.

      a. Routinely and with special tests, 100% have an abnormality.

      b. Chromosome 8 involved.

      c. Good prognosis: t(8,21) M2; inversion of 16 with M4 and eosinophilia.

      d. Poor prognosis: 5q-, 7q-

   3. Clinical factors (poor)

      a. Older; pre-existing preleukemia.

      b. Chemotherapy or toxin-induced; high WBC; poor performance status, metabolic derangements.

3. **Myeloproliferative syndromes**

    a. Clonal disease of pluripotent hematopoietic stem cell with <u>effective</u> increased production of one or more cell types. (This means that the cells work.)

    b. Red cells: Erythrocytosis

    Secondary to increased proliferation of erythroid progenitors <u>or</u> increased production of erythropoietin.

        1. R/O Secondary erythrocytosis

            a. Appropriate: <u>Physiologic</u> attempt by body to increase oxygen carrying capacity in response to tissue hypoxia (congenital cardiac disease with right to left shunt, COPD, carbon monoxide, altitude, high affinity hemoglobinopathy)

            b. <u>Nonphysiologic</u>: due to tumors (hepatoma, renal carcinoma, cerebellar hemangioma), renal cysts.

            c. Diagnosis:

                i. measure erythrocyte mass (increased in all but relative or spurious erythrocytosis)

                ii. measure oxygen saturation; if < 90%, secondary to hypoxemia

                iii. measure CO; increased in smoker's polycythemia

                iv. new use of erythropoietin levels: high in secondary forms, low in polycythemia rubra vera.

                v. rule out high affinity Hgb with abnormal oxyhemoglobin - dissociation curve (P50)

                vi. rule out renal cell with IVP.

2. R/O Relative polycythemia
    (Gaisbock syndrome, spurious, stress erythrocytosis)

    a. Clinical features:

        middle aged men, obese, hypertensive, thromboembolic events in 1/3, smokers (CO-Hbg with decreased plasma volume and increased erythrocyte mass)

    b. Two subsets:

        i. High normal RBC mass

        ii. Low normal plasma volume
            This group gets thromboembolic disease.

    c. Treatment

        i. Underlying disorder

        ii. Phlebotomize #1 and #2 only if cerebral hyperviscous symptoms.

3. Polycythemia rubra vera

    Clonal, myeloproliferative disorder

    a. Clinical features

        Over age 50, insidious onset, hyperviscous symptoms (confusion, headache, blurred vision), bleeding and clotting episodes, circulatory stasis; pruritus, peptic disease secondary to histamine; hyperuricemia and gout, renal stones, splenomegaly.

    b. Lab features

        High leukocyte alkaline phosphatase score, very low plasma and urine erythropoietin, increased vitamin B12 binding protein, absent marrow iron stores (due to frequent GI bleeding).

c. Diagnosis

Triad of erythrocytosis, leukocytosis, thrombocytosis. H/H does not correlate well with RBC mass which must be measured and is increased; r/o chronic hypoxemia, look for presence of splenomegaly.

d. Treatment

Antihistamine
Allopurinol
H2 blockers
Phlebotomy to keep Hct <45, Hgb < 15
Hydroxyurea for increased platelets, painful splenomegaly
Avoid aspirin due to bleeding tendency
If myelofibrosis intervenes, may need to transfuse

e. Natural history

10 year survival
Evolution to myelofibrosis, or acute leukemia (especially if 32P or alkylators used)
Thromboembolic complications.

4. Platelets: Essential thrombocythemia

Least common, clonal disease of pluripotent hematopoietic stem cell.

a. Clinical features

After age 50; may be familial; bleeding; platelet count > 1 million; may develop leukocytosis, splenomegaly, myelofibrosis.

b. Diagnosis

Of exclusion. May be presenting feature of CML (latter has Philadelphia chromosomal marker).

R/O reactive: secondary to iron deficiency anemia, cancer, inflammatory bowel disease, collagen vascular, hemolysis, post splenectomy, rebound after EtOH, rheumatoid arthritis, sickle cell disease.

c. Treatment

No *controlled* study to recommend treatment of increased platelets to decrease risk of thrombosis.

No symptoms, no Rx

If clotting, use hydroxyurea; plateletpheresis is temporary.

Avoid aspirin, as defective platelet function.

d. Natural history

Not well defined. May evolve into acute leukemia, P. vera or myelofibrosis.

5. White cells: Chronic Myelogenous (Granulocytic) Leukemia

Overproduction and malignant transformation of pluripotent stem cell.

a. Clinical features

i. 30% of all leukemia
1 new case/100,000/yr.

ii. Symptoms: malaise, weight loss, fever, night sweats, abdominal fullness (splenomegaly).
Often found incidentally

iii. Related to radiation exposure

b. Lab features

i. Granulocytosis with young cells and mature polys

ii. Eosinophilia, basophilia
Normal to increased platelets.
Low leukocyte alkaline phosphatase stain.

<u>Philadelphia chromosome</u> positive
in bone marrow.
Myelofibrosis in 1/3 (not part
of malignant clone)

iii. Philadelphia chromosome hallmark
t (9q+; 22q-)
Found in precursors of neutrophils, monos, RBC's, platelets.
Not found in lymphocytes.

c. Natural history

i. Usually asymptomatic until well
into course.

ii. Mature polys function, no anemia

iii. "Blast crisis" occurs around 36
months; after 1st year, 25% per
year.
Lymphocytes may be involved in
"crisis" and disease may be
treated like acute <u>lympho-</u>
blastic leukemia. (20% of
cases).
Poor prognosis after blast
crisis.
iv. Median survival from diagnosis
50 months.

d. Treatment

i. Busulfan, hydroxyurea to control
counts.

ii. Interferon may suppress Philadelphia chromosome and control
counts.

iii. Bone marrow transplant in young
patients in chronic phase only
cure.

iv. Supportive care vs. acute leukemia induction when blast
crisis occurs.

C. Disorders of Leukocyte Function (Qualitative Abnormalities)

    1. Decreased chemotaxis - may be a problem in uncontrolled diabetes when glucose > 200.

    2. Decreased killing - chronic granulomatous disease of childhood is the classic.

D. Disorders of Lymphocytes

    1. Too many lymphocytes (usually accumulation of long-lived mature B cells)

        a. Chronic lymphocytic leukemia (marrow end of spectrum from lymphocytic lymphoma)

            1. 50-60 years, male: female 2:1
                Median survival 48 months.

            2. Diagnosis: Persistent monoclonal lymphocytosis. B cells with sIg (IgM, IgD).

                95% are B cells.
                 5% involve T cells.

                Cytogenetic abnormality in 50% with trisomy 12 common.

                Diagnosis made incidentally in 25%.

            3. Rai Classification:

                Stage 0   lymphs 15,000/m3; 25% of patients; survival > 10 years; no treatment.

                Stage I   lymphocytosis; adenopathy; survival 101 months.

                Stage II   hepatosplenomegaly; positive nodes; survival 71 months; need treatment of massive bulky disease.

                Stage III   anemia less than 11g of Hgb; < 2 year survival; need treatment with chlorambucil, prednisone or combination chemotherapy.

Stage IV   thrombocytopenia; < 2 year sur-
            vival; need treatment with
            chlorambucil, prednisone or
            combination chemotherapy. Flu-
            darabine for resistant disease.

May evolve to aggressive lymphoma (Richter syndrome) or myeloma.

4. Hypergammaglobulinemia or hypogammaglobu-
    linemia

    Common
    5% IgM paraprotein
    25% IgG mediated hemolysis
    May need gammaglobulin infusions

5. Chronic T-Cell Lymphocytosis

    Increased T cells; large, granular, sup-
    pressor and natural killer.

    Decreased PMN's, infection.

    Treatment: splenectomy.

b. Lymphocytic lymphoma (<u>tissue end of spectrum
    from CLL</u>)

    See chapter on medical oncology for further
    information.

c. Hairy cell leukemia

    1. New effective treatments with interferon,
        deoxycoformycin so may be important to
        know.

    2. 4th, 5th decade; male; incidental finding
        in 25%.

    3. Symptoms: splenomegaly, infections, ane-
        mia, vasculitis with erythema nodosum,
        cutaneous nodules, visceral involvement.

    4. Mature B cell with "hairs" by phase
        contrast.

        Increased BM reticulin and dry tap despite
        hypercellularity.

Cells with tartrate resistant acid phosphatase (TRAP) are pathognomonic.

Minimal, moderate, massive: Stages I, II, III

    5.   Treatment Stage II, III: splenectomy; interferon; deoxycoformycin; may lead to complete remission.

2.   **Too few** lymphocytes

    a.   Immunodeficiency diseases, congenital

       1.   Bruton's agammaglobulinemia

       2.   IgA deficiency

    b.   Immunodeficiency diseases, acquired

       1.   AIDS

       2.   Common variable hypogammaglobulinemia

3.   **Maturation arrest** of lymphocytes (accumulation of blasts): Immunophenotyping studies of malignant lymphoma show entire spectrum of lymphoid differentiation.

    a.   B cells

       1.   Immunoglobulin (Ig) genes exist as discontinuous segments of DNA (germ-line configuration).

           Must be joined properly to enable synthesis of Ig.

       2.   "Rearrangements" involve separate loci (variable V, diversity D, and joining J response) and the variability allows for diversity of Ig molecules.

       3.   Stages in B cell development can be identified by the particular antigens present on cell surface.

       4.   Undifferentiated lymphoma, B cell, Burkitt type

           Occurs in head and neck in Africa.

Occurs in ovaries/pelvis in America.
C-myc protooncogene translocated from chromosome 8 to loci of immunoglobulin genes; C-myc prevents cellular differentiation.

b. T cells

1. Analogous to B cell differentiation.

2. Genes encoding alpha and beta chains of T cell receptor are rearranged early.

3. <u>Lymphoblastic</u> lymphoma - (Note: different from lympho<u>cytic</u> lymphoma above in D)

a. especially T cell, convoluted, with mediastinal mass in adolescent males; know this symptom complex.

b. HTLV-1 Related

i. Adult T-Cell Leukemia or Lymphoma

ii. Japan, West Indies, Southeastern United States.

iii. Fever, weight loss, increased WBC, increased Ca++.

iv. Late anemia, decreased platelets.

v. Hepatosplenomegaly; skin in 2/3.

4. Disorders of lymphocytes <u>with abnormal proteins</u>

a. Multiple myeloma

1. Neoplastic plasma cell infiltration of marrow, occasionally extramedullary.

2. Solitary plasmacytoma usually of nasopharynx, paranasal sinus; cured with local treatment.

3. Diagnosis of multiple myeloma:

BM plasmacytosis >= 10%
Lytic bone lesions
Serum paraprotein
  IgG 50%, IgA 33%, IgM 5-10%; no protein, 1%
  Urinary light chains 50-75%, not detected by dipstick.
  Hypergammaglobulinemia:

High levels of nonfunctional antibodies.
Increase in suppressor cells leads to decreased antibodies.
Impaired primary antibody response.

4. Clinical consequences

   a. Increased infections.

   b. Bleeding secondary to inactivation of clotting factors and platelets.

   c. Increased serum viscosity = somnolence, coma, bleeding, CHF, visual changes, retinal bleeding.

   d. Increased Ca++ secondary to osteolysis from direct tumor invasion and osteoclast activating factor (OAF).

      Lytic lesions not seen on bone scan secondary to absence of blastic activity.

      Symptoms of increased Ca++: anorexia, nausea, vomiting, constipation, lethargy, renal failure.

      Treatment of increased Ca++: fluids, saline diuresis, steroids, mithramycin, calcitonin, etidronate. Avoid bed rest.

   e. Renal failure:

      Poor prognostic sign.

      Secondary to increased Ca++, increased uric acid, amyloid, toxicity of light chains on tubules.

Contrast agents contraindicated.

Look at urine sediment: light chains or plasma proteins?

f. Pancytopenia: Inhibitory effects of myeloma cells on hematopoiesis. Effects of chemo, RT.

g. Watch for spinal cord compression; sensorimotor neuropathy may occur.

5. Treatment

a. Melphalan and Prednisone x 4 days every 4-6 weeks. 50% response.

b. Interferon for remission maintenance.

c. Erythropoietin for anemia.

d. More aggressive chemo may be better in advanced disease.

e. Median survival 40 months.

f. Secondary leukemia increasing.

b. Waldenstrom macroglobulinemia

1. Older than myeloma patients.

2. Infiltration of marrow, liver, spleen, lymph nodes.

3. No lytic lesions.

4. IgM, hyperviscosity may require plasma-pheresis.

5. Indolent; responds to alkylators.

c. Heavy chain diseases

1. An incomplete gammaglobulin is produced.

2. Alpha heavy chain disease: lymphoid areas of GI tract; malabsorption; diarrhea; Near East, North Africa.

           3. Gamma disease: Presents as lymphoma (nodes, hepatosplenomegaly, fever, weight loss).

           4. Mu disease: Variant of CLL with increased spleen, decreased nodes.

           5. Responds poorly.

    d. "Benign" monoclonal gammopathy (BMG) or monoclonal gammopathy of undetermined significance (MGUS)

           1. If no monoclonality, no neoplasia.

           2. BMG common, > 3% persons > 70 years, usually IgG.

           3. Benign features: IgG < 3 grams, normal Ig production; absent marrow plasmacytosis, no lytic lesions; normal Ca++.

           4. If gammopathy search for plasmacytoma.

           5. Other neoplasms with paraproteins: renal, lung, GI.

           6. Infections with paraproteins: TB, hepatitis; cirrhosis.

           7. Follow-up every three months for one year, then annually.

           8. If changes, re-evaluate.

           9. Study of natural history: 241 patients with 10 year follow-up. Neoplasis developed in 19% at median 8-10 years after diagnosis of BMG.

5. Genetics of leukemia

Chronic myelogenous leukemia t(9;22). Know this one!

Acute myelogenous leukemia trisomy 8 or t(8;21)

Acute promyelocytic leukemia M3 t(15;17)

Acute myeloid leukemia without differentiation M2 (t8;21) associated with good prognosis

Leukemias 5 q - or 7 q - : poor prognosis.

Myelodysplasia 5 q -

Immunoglobulin genes on 14, 2, 22

Burkitt lymphoma and L3 leukemia t(8;14) or t8;2 or 22)

Chronic lymphocytic leukemia trisomy 12, t(11;14)

Multiple myeloma t(11;14), as CLL

Follicular small cleaved cell lymphoma (poorly differentiated, nodular) t(14;18).

V. DISORDERS OF PLATELETS

A. Thrombocytopenia

    1. Due to bone marrow failure (decreased production)

        a. aplastic anemia

        b. drug-induced

            1. chemotherapy

            2. alcohol

            3. carbenicillin

        c. myelodysplasia

    2. Due to peripheral destruction (increased production)

        a. autoimmune

            1. lupus

            2. ITP

            3. AIDS/HIV

        b. hypersplenism

        c. drug-induced

            1. heparin

        2. thiazides

        3. quinidine

    d. disseminated intravascular coagulation

B. Thrombocytosis

    1. Reactive

        a. stress

        b. infection

        c. surgery

        d. iron deficiency

        e. sickle cell disease

        f. malignancy

        g. rheumatoid arthritis

    2. Malignant

        a. essential thrombocytosis

        b. other myeloproliferative

            1. polycythemia vera

            2. chronic granulocytic (myelogenous) leukemia

        c. Treat with hydroxyurea

        d. Disorders of platelet function - bleeding time will be prolonged in <u>both</u> qualitative and quantitative platelet disorders.

            1. Qualitative platelet defects

                a. Von Willebrand's - prolonged PTT, abnormal ristocetin aggregation. Mild mucosal bleeding.

                b. aspirin - prolonged bleeding time.

     c. myelodysplasia - acquired; may need platelet transfusion if bleeding, regardless of platelet number.

   2. Quantitative platelet defects

     a. < 100,000, transfuse for surgical procedures

     b. < 20,000, risk of spontaneous bleeding

     c. transfusions commonly given in acute leukemia prophylactically when < 20,000 (controversial in era of cost containment).

   3. Platelet thought to have a major role in initiating events of myocardial infarction, thrombotic thrombocytopenic purpura.

VI. QUESTIONS

1. The common causes of microcytic hypochromic anemia are

   a. iron deficiency anemia
   b. thalassemia
   c. B12 and folate deficiency
   d. alcoholism
   e. (a) and (b) only

2. Salmonella osteomyelitis is a classic association of

   a. sickle cell anemia
   b. B12 and folate deficiency
   c. autoimmune hemolytic anemia
   d. iron deficiency anemia

3. Causes of disseminated intravascular coagulation (DIC) include

   a. sepsis
   b. endothelial damage
   c. burn patients
   d. obstetrical castastrophies
   e. all of the above

4. Symptoms of the hyperviscosity syndrome include (multiple true-false)

   a. blurred vision
   b. headaches
   c. weakness
   d. dyspnea
   e. gangrene

5. The initial treatment of in-hospital, severe, symptomatic hypercalcemia in a cancer patient is

   a. normal saline hydration
   b. furosemide
   c. steroids
   d. phosphates

6. The classic laboratory findings in iron deficiency are

   a. low MCV, low iron, low total iron binding capacity, low ferritin
   b. low MCV, low iron, high total iron binding capacity, low ferritin
   c. low MCV, low iron, low total iron binding capacity, high ferritin
   d. high MCV, low iron, low total iron binding capacity, high ferritin

7. Iron deficiency and thalassemia minor share all but one of the following

   a. microcytosis
   b. hypochromia
   c. poikilocytosis
   d. low serum iron
   e. low ferritin

8. Patients with sickle cell anemia are at risk for which of the following (multiple true-false)

   a. pneumococcus infections
   b. salmonella infections
   c. hemosiderosis
   d. aseptic necrosis of bone
   e. malaria

9. All of the following are features of thrombotic thrombocytopenic purpura EXCEPT

   a. fever
   b. renal failure
   c. hemolytic anemia
   d. diabetes
   e. thrombocytopenia

10. One of the following statements about autoimmune thrombocytopenic purpura is false

   a. The spleen is markedly enlarged.
   b. The bone marrow contains many megakaryocytes.
   c. The spleen is hot on nuclear scan.
   d. Petechiae are seen in dependent locations and mucous membranes.
   e. Platelet transfusion rarely results in significant rise in platelet count.

11. A young man presents with a second episode of spontaneous deep vein thrombosis. Before heparin is begun, all of the following tests are indicated EXCEPT

   a. protein S level
   b. protein C level
   c. CT scan of abdomen looking for cancer
   d. antithrombin III level
   e. partial thromboplastin time

12. Thrombocytosis is associated with which of the following (multiple true-false)

   a. chronic myelogenous leukemia
   b. acute myelogenous leukemia
   c. polycythemia rubra vera
   d. iron deficiency
   e. rheumatoid arthritis
   f. systemic lupus erythematosus
   g. essential thrombocythemia

13. A 69-year-old black male has had a myelodysplastic syndrome for two years requiring blood transfusions and antibiotics for frequent infections due to neutropenia. He presents now with fever, increasing numbers of blasts (50%), skin petechiae, necrotic material in his nares, and space occupying lesions of liver on CT scan. His clinical picture is most compatible with

a. aplastic anemia
b. paroxysmal nocturnal hemoglobinuria
c. acute myelofibrosis
d. acute leukemia with disseminated aspergillosis
e. metastatic carcinoma of unknown primary

VII. **ANSWERS**

1. e

2. a

3. e

4. a-True; b-True; c-True; d-True; e-False

5. a

6. b

7. e

8. a-True; b-True; c-True; d-True; e-False

9. d

10. a

11. c

12. a-True; b-False; c-True; d-True; e-True; f-False; g-True

13. d

I. COMMON SOLID TUMORS

A. Lung Cancer

1. Role of smoking and other cofactors - smoking is major risk factor. Asbestos exposure is cocarcinogenic with smoking. Pulmonary fibrosis is a minor risk factor.

2. Small cell - considered metastatic at diagnosis. Treated with chemotherapy primarily and radiation. Commonly was given brain irradiation prophylactically.

3. Nonsmall cell - large cell, squamous, adenocarcinoma behave similarly. Treated with surgery if possible, radiation if not. Not very chemo sensitive.

B. Breast Cancer

1. Screening - baseline mammogram age 35-40, annual mammogram after 50

2. Role of genetics and other cofactors:

Increased risk with

    Breast Ca in mother, sister
    Breast Ca in contralateral breast
        (or ipsilateral if breast tissue remains)
    Nulliparity
    Obesity
    High fat diet
    Radiation to chest
    One type of fibrocystic disease:
        atypical hyperplasia

3. Treatment - End results are similar for radical mastectomy, modified radical mastectomy, and lumpectomy or quadrantectomy with irradiation. The key concept is

    a. to remove the tumor.

    b. to either remove the remaining breast tissue or to radiate it to prevent new focus in that breast.

    c. to sample axillary nodes to determine one's likelihood of occult systemic disease.

    d. to treat systemically if nodes are positive with either chemotherapy if premenopausal or tamoxifen if postmenopausal.

    e. Adjuvant treatment and its rationale - axillary lymph nodes containing tumor are a marker for systemic disease requiring further systemic therapy. Premenopausal women generally get chemotherapy for 6 months. Postmenopausal women generally get hormonal therapy with tamoxifen for 5 years.

C. Rectal Cancer (See Gastroenterology Section)

D. Colon Cancer (See Gastroenterology Section)

1. Therapy for metastatic disease - 5 FU/Leucovorin, 5 FU/interferon, surgical resection of liver metastases if feasible.

E. Prostate Cancer

1. Screening: use of rectal exam, ultrasound, and prostate specific antigen - These are used singly and in combination. Their role is not yet known.

2. Staging

Stage A	found incidentally on TURP
Stage B	nodule within prostate
Stage C	outside capsule
Stage D(1)	lymph nodes adjacent to prostate
Stage D(2)	bony or distant metastases

3. Treatment

   a. Surgery - nerve sparing surgery done on early lesions (A,B) to maintain potency

   b. Radiation therapy - for C lesions

   c. Hormonal manipulation: orchiectomy, diethyl-stilbestrol, or leuprolide, (gonadotropin stimulating hormone analog), plus flutamide (antiandrogen) for D lesions. This treats the gland and distant metastases.

II. **MEDICALLY CURABLE CANCERS**

A. Acute lymphoblastic leukemia - more common in children and adolescents.

   1. Set the stage as a model for a medically curable cancer

   2. Use of noncross-resistant drugs in a sequence for a defined length of time

   3. CNS intrathecal prophylaxis, as the CNS is a "sanctuary site" due to inability of drugs to cross blood-brain barrier.

   4. Bone marrow transplant: homologous and autologous used after relapse.

   5. Chromosomal markers (see above "Genetics of Leukemia")

B. Lymphomas

1. <u>Cell type</u> and <u>pattern</u> (diffuse or aggressive vs. follicular or nodular, indolent) more important than stage.

(New) Working Formulation	(Old) Rappaport Classification	Markers	Survival
Low grade follicular, small cleaved cell	Nodular, poorly differentiated lymphocytic	B	7.2 years
Intermediate grade diffuse, large cell	Diffuse histiocytic	B or none	1.5 years (but may be curable)
High grade large cell immunoblastic	Diffuse histiocytic	B, T, or neither	1.3 years (may be curable)
lymphoblastic (convoluted cell)	Lymphoblastic	T or none	2.0 years
small non-cleaved cell	Undifferentiated, Burkitt	B	0.7 years

2. Note how lymphomas relate to other hematologic diseases.

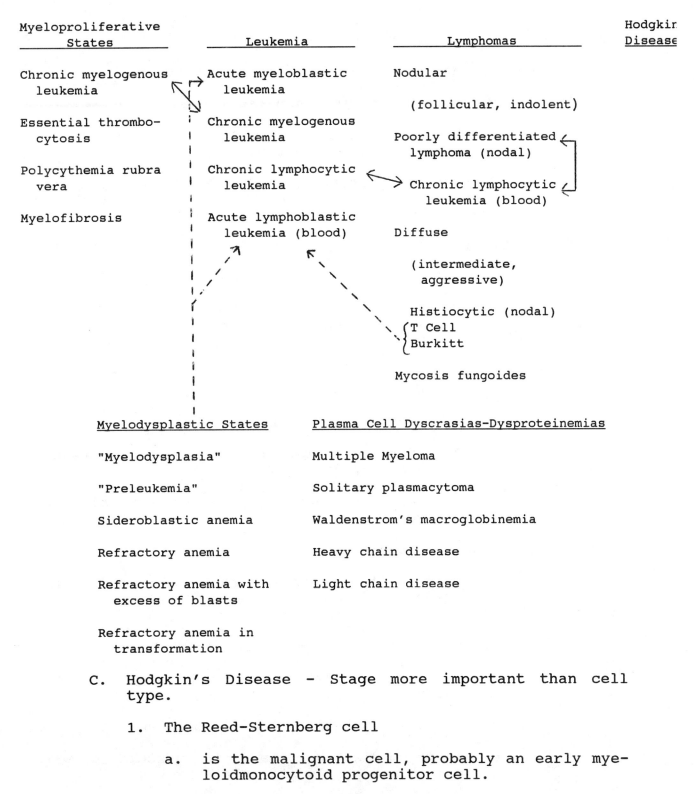

Myeloproliferative States	Leukemia	Lymphomas	Hodgkin Disease
Chronic myelogenous leukemia	Acute myeloblastic leukemia	Nodular (follicular, indolent)	
Essential thrombocytosis	Chronic myelogenous leukemia	Poorly differentiated lymphoma (nodal)	
Polycythemia rubra vera	Chronic lymphocytic leukemia	Chronic lymphocytic leukemia (blood)	
Myelofibrosis	Acute lymphoblastic leukemia (blood)	Diffuse (intermediate, aggressive)	
		Histiocytic (nodal) T Cell Burkitt	
		Mycosis fungoides	

Myelodysplastic States	Plasma Cell Dyscrasias-Dysproteinemias
"Myelodysplasia"	Multiple Myeloma
"Preleukemia"	Solitary plasmacytoma
Sideroblastic anemia	Waldenstrom's macroglobinemia
Refractory anemia	Heavy chain disease
Refractory anemia with excess of blasts	Light chain disease
Refractory anemia in transformation	

C. Hodgkin's Disease - Stage more important than cell type.

    1. The Reed-Sternberg cell

        a. is the malignant cell, probably an early myeloidmonocytoid progenitor cell.

b. may be from antigen presenting dendritic reticulum cells in parafollicular zone of node.

c. found in mono, other tumors.

d. needed for diagnosis; not pathognomonic.

e. node biopsy (not aspirate) needed.

f. histologic subtype less important than stage for treatment selection.

2. Cure is now possible in 75% - 80% of all patients with the <u>extent of disease</u> being very important in selection of therapy and prognosis.

3. Histologic type is less important prognostically due to excellent therapy.

4. Staging:

    I - Single lymph node area
   II - Two or more areas on the same side of the diaphragm.
 III - Nodes on both sides of the diaphragm.
  IV - Extra-nodal tissues or organs.

    A   Represents absence of symptoms.

    B   Represents presence of symptoms of fever, night sweats, weight loss.

    E   Represents extra-lymphatic extension by contiguity.

5. Staging laparotomy

a. Done in Stage I or II patients to confirm the <u>absence</u> of disease in the abdomen.

b. Lymphangiogram important - should do in early stage disease if negative results will change treatment (ie: chemotherapy for advanced disease changed to radiation therapy (RT) for early disease).

c. 1/3 will upstage, 1/5 will downstage.

d. Large mediastinal mass is associated with anesthesia complications at surgery.

6. Treatment:

    a. Stages I and II-A

        1. treated with extended field radiation <u>except</u> when they have very bulky disease where chemotherapy may be added in.

        2. If relapse after RT, can be salvaged with chemo but increased second malignancies; so, early but high risk patients may need initial combined treatment.

    b. Stage II-B is treated with combined modality therapy (involved field radiotherapy and combination chemotherapy).

    c. Stage III-A disease treatment is controversial.

    d. Stages III-B and IV disease are treated with combination chemotherapy.

7. Chemotherapy

    a. MOPP (Mustard, Oncovin, Procarbazine, Prednisone)

    b. ABVD (Adriamycin, Bleomycin, Vinblastine, DTIC)

    c. or alternating these two combinations.

    d. Principles: use full doses and per schedule.

8. Complications of therapy:

    a. Radiation-induced heart disease (pericardial and coronary) occurs late, around 10 years.

    b. Hypothyroidism.

    c. Sterility.

    d. Osteoporosis in females due to lack of estrogen.

    e. <u>Second malignancies</u>, with acute nonlymphocytic leukemia being the most serious, usually in patients receiving both radiation therapy and chemotherapy.

f. Immune Defects

1. Cell mediated, especially in advanced disease, and persists for years: TB, virus, pneumocystis.

2. Humoral immunity suppressed secondary to treatment.

3. Splenectomy for staging predisposes to pneumococcus and H flu. Give Pneumovax pre-splenectomy.

D. Testicular: Seminoma, Nonseminoma

1. High risk - Patients with cryptorchid testes: both the undescended and the descended testis

2. Markers - HCG and alpha fetoprotein are elevated, primarily in nonseminomas; are very sensitive markers for disease.

3. Surgery - Primary treatment. If markers remain increased post op orchidectomy, a retroperitoneal node dissection may be done.

4. Chemotherapy - Nonseminomas are curable with chemotherapy, even when widely metastatic.

5. Some nonseminomas (teratocarcinomas) may transform to benign teratomas with chemotherapy. If masses remain and markers are normal, surgical resection needs to be done for diagnosis.

6. Seminomas are radiosensitive. Radiation therapy is generally given to areas of known disease and one level higher (ex: to retroperitoneal nodes and mediastinum for known disease in the former).

E. Acute Non-Lymphocytic Leukemia (Acute Myelogenous Leukemia)

1. Proliferation of cells arrested at a primitive stage.

2. Symptoms of bleeding, infection, anemia (marrow failure).

3. See section Disorders of Leukocytes, Hematology Chapter

4. Treatment:

a. Goal: to decrease leukemic cells so normal hematopoiesis can resume.

    1. Cytarabine, Daunorubicin
        < 70 years, complete remission 55-60%
        < 40 years, complete remission 70%

    2. Use heparin with FAB M3 to prevent DIC

    3. Once complete remission, may give monthly treatment x 8 at reduced doses or 2-4 more courses of remission induction doses.

        Median remission duration for complete responders 18-24 months; 30-50% patients stay in complete remission 3 years.

        5-20% mortality from treatment.

    4. CNS prophylax M4,5.

    5. If relapse, poor prognosis.

    6. Treat early unless:

        a. severe infection.

        b. metabolic derangements (renal failure, increased uric acid, increased LFT's).

        c. poor performance status (bedridden).

        d. elderly > 70 - consider low-dose therapy; consider supportive care.

5. Transfuse when platelets < 20,000 or if febrile, < 30,000.

6. Treat with antibiotics when febrile (after work-up). Use aminoglycoside and antipseudomonal PCN or if allergic, 3rd generation cephalosporin.

    If fever persists without documented bacterial infections, add antifungal. Consider pneumocystis.

7. Granulocyte transfusion indicated only if severe neutropenia (< 500 x 10^6) and bacteremic or unresponsive skin and/or oral infection. Can cause adult respiratory distress syndrome, especially with Amphotericin B.

8. Prevent metabolic complications - use allopurinol, fluids, alkali phosphate binders. May get increased K.

9. Hyperleukocytosis is an emergency. Can get decreased pO2, CNS bleed. Leukapheresis, chemotherapy (1 gram Cytoxan IV, or hydroxyurea 5 grams po) or whole brain irradiation.

10. CNS leukemia in 3-5% as opposed to 25% of acute lymphoblastic leukemia.

F. Acute Lymphoblastic Leukemia

1. 15% adult leukemia

2. Peroxidase negative blasts

3. French American British (FAB) categories:

   L1 small, homogeneous, big nucleus, small nucleoli

   L2 larger, pleomorphic, prominent nucleolus; increases with age

   L3 large, vacuolated cytoplasm, large nucleus and nucleolus; leukemic counterpart of Burkitt lymphoma t(8:14) translocation

4. Immunologic categories: (4 major)

   a. B cell lineage (65% of cases)
      React with BA-1 or CALLA
      Nonreactive with T cell markers

   b. T cell (15%) Tdt (+) ("terminal transferase")
      All react with anti-T antibodies
      1/3 E rosette (+); Male, mediastinal adeno-
         pathy
      (Remember from Hematology chapter?)

   c. Non B, non T (9%)

   d. React with myeloid antigens.

5. Good prognostic signs

   FAB L1 type
   CALLA positive
   Young age
   Modal chromosome > 50
   Pre B phenotype
   Low WBC
   No extramedullary disease

6. Bad prognostic signs

   FAB L3 (Burkitt-like)
   Presence of Ph chromosome
   Chromosomal translocations
   CNS disease, mediastinal disease
   High WBC
   B cell or T cell, myeloid positive

7. Adult disease:

   CALLA negative
   FAB L2 common

8. Treatment:

   a. Vincristine,   Prednisone,   Daunorubicin,
      L-asparaginase.

   b. Intrathecal MTX, cranial radiation for CNS
      prophylaxis.

   c. If complete remission, maintenance with 6 MP
      and MTX for 3 years.

   d. Median duration of complete remission 16
      months. 20% in complete remission at 5 years.

   e. Consolidation treatment important.

   f. Pneumocystis common.

G. Bone Marrow Transplantation in Acute Leukemia

   1. Factors: Age > 35 years, and first remission, 1
      year mortality > 50%; < 20 years, 1 year mortality
      < 20%

Better results when done in remission and in the young

Organ function

2. Preferred treatment for patients < 20 years, HLA identical match: > 70% long-term disease-free survival.

3. For patients > 30 years, chemotherapy then transplant in early relapse.

4. Treatment of choice for patient with several relapses.

5. Mismatched donor studies and autologous transplant studies ongoing.

6. Less effective for ALL than ANLL.

H. Antineoplastic Agents

Memorize, learn the exceptions

Drug	Mode of Action	Major Side/Effect	Myelo-suppression at Usual Doses
Cyclophosphamide	alkylator	hemorrhagic cystitis	yes
Doxorubicin	anthracycline antibiotic (alkylator)	cardiotoxicity	yes
Platinum	heavy metal (alkylator)	renal toxicity	mild
Bleomycin	antibiotic (scission)	pulmonary fibrosis	no
Methotrexate	folate antagonist	liver fibrosis	yes
6 Mercaptopurine	folate antagonist	cirrhosis	yes
5 Fluorouracil	folate antagonist	diarrhea, mucositis	yes

Drug	Mode of Action	Major Side/Effect	Myelo-suppression at Usual Doses
Etoposide	mitotic inhibitor	myelosuppression	yes
Vincristine	tubule poison	neurotoxicity	no
Vinblastine	tubule poison	myalgia	yes

III. PARANEOPLASTIC SYNDROMES

Syndrome	Associated Cancer
SIADH	small cell lung cancer
Cushing's	small cell lung cancer
Eaton Lambert	small cell lung cancer
Ectopic PTH	nonsmall cell lung cancer (this is the exception) esophageal renal cell
Polycythemia	renal cell hepatoma cerebellar astrocytoma
Hypercoagulable state	mucin-producing adenocarcinomas: lung, stomach, pancreas, prostate with activated factor X
DIC	acute promyelocytic leukemia (FAB M3)
Dermatomyositis	colon, stomach, lung
Hypoglycemia	islet cell tumor retroperitoneal sarcomas
Diarrhea	VIPomas

IV. **QUESTIONS**

1. A 65-year-old black male veteran has a history of heavy alcohol and cigarette abuse. He is at risk for which of the following? (multiple true-false)

    a. bladder cancer
    b. neurofibrosarcoma
    c. laryngeal cancer
    d. lung cancer
    e. pharyngeal cancer
    f. esophageal cancer
    g. prostate cancer

2. The work-up of a patient with a prostate nodule include(s) (multiple true-false)

    a. PSA
    b. prostatic ultrasound
    c. chest CT scan
    d. bone scan
    e. CT brain scan

3. A classic example of co-carcinogenicity is

    a. dietary fat and familial polyposis
    b. chest wall irradiation and nulliparity
    c. asbestos and cigarette smoke
    d. sunlight and fair complexion
    e. papilloma virus and early sexual intercourse

4. A 62-year-old white male was diagnosed with gastric lymphoma, diffuse large-cell type, and chemotherapy was begun. Two weeks post treatment he developed severe abdominal pain, a rigid abdomen, and absent bowel sounds. Upright film showed free air. What happened?

    a. typhlitis from neutropenia from chemotherapy
    b. vincristine related autonomic neuropathy of bowel
    c. perforation of stomach from rapidly shrinking tumor
    d. stress-related gastritis
    e. gallstone ileus

5. Which of the following cancers is least likely to have associated hypercalcemia?

    a. breast cancer
    b. myeloma
    c. large-cell lung cancer
    d. small-cell lung cancer
    e. renal cell

6. A patient presents with dyspnea and facial, neck, and hand swelling. A right upper lobe mass is present on chest film. The most likely explanation for symptoms is

    a. anemia
    b. cancer-related glomerulonephritis
    c. heart failure
    d. superior vena cava syndrome
    e. inferior vena cava obstruction

7. A patient was treated for small-call lung cancer with chemotherapy ten days ago. He presents now with fever to 103°, malaise, and pallor. His Hgb is 7.9 g, his WBC is 0.3, and platelets are 60,000. The most important aspect of treatment is

    a. transfusion of red cells
    b. transfusion of white cells
    c. transfusion of platelets
    d. initiation of intravenous fluids
    e. initiation of antibiotics

8. A 70-year-old black male was treated with radiation therapy for prostate cancer. After 5 weeks, he began to complain of dysuria. Urine was positive for hemoglobin and culture negative. He likely had

    a. hemorrhagic cystitis from cyclophosphamide
    b. pyelonephritis
    c. ureteral stone
    d. recurrence of prostate cancer
    e. radiation cystitis

9. A 25-year-old otherwise healthy white female complained of a two-month history of right cervical mass. A pre-biopsy chest x-ray revealed a mediastinal mass. Biopsy revealed large cells with double mirror image nuclei and prominent nucleoli. The diagnosis is

   a. nodular sclerosing Hodgkin's disease
   b. squamous cell carcinoma of the base of the tongue
   c. cat scratch disease
   d. bronchial cleft cyst
   e. T cell lymphoma

10. A 53-year-old alcoholic smoker presented with a large right cervical mass and pain in his throat. A likely diagnosis is

   a. nodular sclerosing Hodgkin's disease
   b. squamous cell carcinoma of the base of the tongue
   c. cat scratch disease
   d. bronchial cleft cyst
   e. T cell lymphoma

11. A 17-year-old black male basketball player presented with fevers, a right cervical mass, and a chest film showing a mediastinal mass. His WBC was 84,000 with 60% blasts. A likely diagnosis is

   a. nodular sclerosing Hodgkin's disease
   b. squamous cell carcinoma of the base of the tongue
   c. cat scratch disease
   d. bronchial cleft cyst
   e. T cell lymphoma

V. ANSWERS

1. a-True; b-False; c-True; d-True; e-True; f-True; g-True

2. a-True; b-True; c-False; d-True; e-False

3. c

4. c

5. d

6. d

7. e

8. e

9. a

10. b

11. e

I. <u>DIABETES, INSULIN DEPENDENT, JUVENILE ONSET, TYPE I</u>

Usually in younger patients, < 40 years, 10% of all diabetics.

A. Etiologic Theories

Autoimmune, viral. Onset possibly related to pancreatic infection with mumps, Coxsackie, rubella viruses. Early antibodies to islet cells are found. Thyroid and other auto antibodies may be present.

B. Chromosomal Predisposition

HLA types: specific HLA's on short arm of chromosome 6, HLA DR3, DW3, DR4, B8, B15, D locus more important. 50% concordance rate in identical twins.

C. Diabetic Ketoacidosis (DKA)

Most children present with DKA. They are sick a short time (days) before seeking medical care.

1. Pathogenesis of DKA: Double-pronged

a. Insulin lack, increased lipolysis, increased plasma free fatty acids, increased liver fatty acids, <u>increased ketones</u>.

b. Glucagon excess, decreased malonyl COA, increased carnitine acyltransferase, <u>increased ketones</u>.

2. Diagnosis:

a. Symptoms: anorexia, nausea, vomiting, often abdominal pain (common in acidosis, not just

DKA), polyuria. May have fever, history of recent infection, surgery or stress.

b. Signs: Hypotension, tachycardia, poor skin turgor, Kussmaul (deep and regular, frequent) respirations, lethargy.

c. Lab: blood glucose very high, Occasionally > 1,000. Very low bicarb, low pCO_2, K+ may be high, creatinine usually up, serum and urine acetone positive (the former in a dilution > 1:1)

3. Management: saline, regular insulin, replace potassium as needed. Treat any infection. Correction should take hours. Brain edema and seizures occur when therapy is too fast; death can occur when too slow.

D. Therapy

Diabetic diet and snacks. Split dose insulin for "tight" control. Home glucose monitoring important. Keep Hgb Al-C less than 9.

E. Complications

Tight control does not necessarily prevent these:

1. Retinopathy - Early microaneurysms (dot hemorrhages), flame hemorrhages. Neovascularization (proliferative) needs laser therapy, very common cause of blindness but is preventable. Do not use heparin in patients with proliferative retinopathy. Retinopathy occurs after ten years of diabetes.

2. Neuropathy:

a. Sensory

1. Painful burning of feet.

2. Loss of sensation leads to unnoticed trauma, ulcers, infection.

b. Mononeuritis multiplex (self-limited).

1. Cranial nerve palsy, especially 6th and 3rd. Pupils spared and continue to react, differentiating from some other problems.

        2.   Femoral nerve amyotrophy (pain and weak-
            ness of thigh)

    c. Autonomic

        1.   Orthostasis

        2.   Gastroparesis

        3.   Diarrhea

3. Nephropathy: common cause of end stage renal failure. Glucose control gets easier in renal failure as insulin is not excreted/metabolized by the damaged kidney.

4. Vascular disease:

    a. small vessel disease leads to ulcers of feet, cardiomyopathy, neuropathy (as vessels nourishing nerves are involved), multi-infarction dementia.

    b. large vessel disease leads to MI, CVA, claudication with painful ischemia of feet and legs.

II. DIABETES, NONINSULIN DEPENDENT, NONKETOSIS PRONE, MATURITY ONSET, TYPE II

A. Etiology

    1. Hereditable influence - familial; 100% concordance rate in identical twins. Not HLA related however.

    2. Obesity - Maintenance of ideal body weight and exercise may help prevent in patients at risk.

B. Diagnosis

Fasting blood sugar > 140 mg/dl. 2 hour pc blood sugars > 200. Glucose tolerance test is too sensitive and is not used.

Special consideration: pregnancy-induced, steroid-induced (these patients may require short-term therapy)

"Chemical" diabetics or glucose intolerance - only 30%
progress to overt diabetes

C. Management

1. Diabetic education by nurse, dietician

2. Diet - cornerstone of management. Practically it
    is very hard to achieve weight loss.

3. Exercise - data suggest exercise may forestall
    onset.

4. Oral agents - glyburide and glipizide very
    popular.

    As with older agents, beware of hypoglycemia in
    elderly and renal failure. Know phenformin caused
    lactic acidosis (now off the market) and chlor-
    propamide causes SIADH.

5. Insulin - theory of insulin excess which accele-
    rates atherogenesis. Some patients cannot be
    controlled with diet and oral agents. Combining
    the latter with insulin is controversial; some
    give oral agent in AM, insulin at night.

6. Home glucose monitoring very important

D. Complications

Similar to those seen in Type I diabetes. Generally
less severe, not as predictable.

1. Retinopathy

2. Neuropathy

3. Nephropathy - ACE inhibitors are used to prevent
    glomerular hypertension in patients with micro-
    albuminuria, thought to be precursor to renal
    failure.

4. Vascular disease

    a. ASHD - these patients usually succumb to heart
        disease. Treat other risk factors as well as
        diabetes.

b. Peripheral vascular disease - be careful not to induce renal failure with contrast agents used to diagnose vascular disease!

c. Cerebrovascular disease

E. Prevention

By maintaining ideal body weight and exercise.

III. **THYROID DISEASE**

A. Thyroid Function Tests

New nomenclature: free T4 and "sensitive" TSH which can measure low values are the tests of choice.

Disorder	Free T4	TSH	Free T3
Thyroid gland failure	Decreased	Increased	
Thyrotoxicosis	Decreased	Decreased < 0.1 mU/L	
"Sick euthyroid" (mild to moderate)	Normal or increased	Normal	
"Very sick euthyroid" (severe [ICU])	Decreased	May be increased with recovery	
T3 toxicosis	Normal	Decreased	Increased (use only to rule
Hypothalamic or pituitary related hypothyroidism	Decreased	Decreased	in this diag- nosis)
Dopamine or large dose steroid therapy			

B. Autoimmune

1. Hashimoto's thyroiditis - Lymphocytic infiltration of gland.

a. Symptoms - as in hypothyroidism. Common in adolescents and females. Associated with other autoimmune diseases: diabetes, pernicious anemia, lupus.

    b. Signs - common cause for goiter. Associated anti-thyroglobulin antibody and antimicrosomal antibodies. With time, increasing hypothyroidism.

    c. Management - needs thyroid replacement.

    d. Genetic predisposition - thyroid disease tends to run in families.

2. Graves' disease - more common in females.

    a. Symptoms - weight loss despite good appetite, heat intolerance, increased energy, increased sweating, palpitations, collar tightness or dysphagia due to goiter, diplopia, loose stools.

    b. Signs - tachycardia, injected conjunctivae, goiter with bruit, "velvet" skin, splenomegaly (rare), proptosis, lid lag, exophthalmos, lymphocytosis, low cholesterol.

    c. Management - radioactive iodine, thyroidectomy, beta blockers, antithyroid drugs.

    d. Genetic predisposition - thyroid disease tends to run in families; associated autoimmune diseases

3. Toxic multinodular goiter.

    a. Arises in long-standing simple goiter; seen in elderly.

    b. Weakness and wasting are common. May have prominent cardiovascular symptoms.

    c. TRH stimulation test shows subnormal or absent TSH response.

    d. Radioactive iodine treatment of choice.

4. Thyroid storm (rare).

    a. Increase in signs and symptoms of thyrotoxicosis.

    b. Precipitation by surgery, sepsis, stress.

      c.   Fever, coma, confusion, agitation, tachycardia, vomiting, shock.

      d.   Treat with antithyroid drugs, iodine, beta blockers, Decadron, fluids.

C. Thyroid Nodule

Usually a cold nodule.

1. Diagnosis

      a.   physical exam (rarely symptomatic)

      b.   scans - patients who have had head and neck irradiation are at risk for nodules and cancer.

2. Management - need to establish if a cold nodule is malignant (hot nodules are not) by fine needle biopsy or excision. Suppress TSH with levothyroxine.

D. Thyroid Cancer

1. Papillary - most common. Increased incidence after head and neck irradiation. Recurs locally in neck. Responds to radioactive iodine as treatment. Metastasizes to bone. Indolent over years.

2. Follicular - second most common, more aggressive than papillary.

3. Medullary carcinoma - Associated with other endocrine adenomas. Common exam question: Patient found to have increased calcitonin and medullary carcinoma of thyroid. Noted to be sporadically hypertensive and sweats a lot. You need to look for a pheochromocytoma. Also to check family members with serum calcitonins, may need to stimulate with pentagastrin.

4. Anaplastic - rapidly fatal over weeks.

5. Lymphoma - usually large cell (histiocytic)

E. Medical Considerations in Hypothyroidism

1. Symptoms of hypothyroidism - fatigue, inability to concentrate, hoarseness, slowness of thought, weight gain, cold intolerance, constipation.

2. Signs - thickened skin (pretibial myxedema), coarse hair, scratchy voice, mental dullness, slowed DTR's, loss of lateral eyebrows, subnormal body temperature, pleural and pericardial effusions, low amplitude EKG.

3. Lab - low serum T4, elevated TSH (must have functioning pituitary). Can have low TSH if pituitary diseased. Cholesterol high.

4. Institution of thyroid replacement - must start low, go slow to avoid precipitation of cardiac symptoms in most medical patients. Treatment causes exacerbation of coronary artery disease; so much so that thyroid ablation used to be a treatment for angina.

5. Failure to wean from ventilator post op; consider this along with maximizing other metabolic and nutritional parameters.

6. Failure to thrive postoperatively - fluid retention, slow convalescence, no energy.

7. Concomitant adrenal insufficiency is very common so think about this!

IV. **PARATHYROID DISEASE**

A. Differential Diagnosis of Hypercalcemia

1. Hyperparathyroidism - most common

2. Lytic bone lesions - secondary to malignancy

3. Ectopic PTH

4. Immobilization, dehydration

5. Vitamin D toxicity

6. Calcium-containing antacids

7. Addison's disease

8. Hyperthyroidism

9. Granulomatous diseases

B. Symptoms of Hypercalcemia

   1. Bone disease

      a. Pain

      b. Cysts

      c. Osteoporosis

   2. Digestive symptoms

      a. Gastritis

      b. Indigestion

      c. Reflux

      d. Gas

      e. Peptic ulcer disease

      f. Constipation

   3. Renal disease

      a. Stones (moans, _stones_, bones, and groans)

      b. Decreased creatinine clearance

   4. Neuro-psychiatric symptoms - confusion, lethargy, irritability, weakness.

C. Diagnosis of Parathyroid Adenoma

   1. Increased calcium

   2. Increased PTH in the presence of high calcium

   3. Localization by MRI

D. Treatment of Parathyroid Adenoma

   1. Neck exploration - after MRI. Can be a cause for vocal cord paralysis if recurrent laryngeal nerve damaged.

2. Failed exploration - if hypercalcemia recurs post op, consider venous sampling for PTH to aid in localizing.

3. Chest exploration - substernal thyroids and para-thyroids exist!

4. Postoperative hypocalcemia - may require intensive monitoring and replacement.

E. Secondary Hyperparathyroidism

Simply, renal failure leads to renal leak of calcium and hypocalcemia. Parathyroid compensates by produc-tion of PTH and calcium is leached out of bones.

F. Tertiary Hyperparathyroidism

Renal failure leads to renal leak of calcium and hypo-calcemia. Parathyroid becomes autonomously hyper-active, adenomatous.

G. Multiple Endocrine Neoplasia

Involved Site	Type I (Wermer syndrome)	Type IIa (Sipple syndrome)	Type IIb (worse progno-sis than IIa)
Parathyroid	Tumors or hyperplasia	Hyperplasia in 50%	Rare
Pancreas	Insulinoma, gastrinoma, glucagonoma		
Pituitary	Acromegaly or Cushing's		
Pheochromocytoma		Occ bilateral, extraadrenal	As IIa
Mucosal neuroma			Multiple
Medullary CA thyroid		Increased calcitonin, ACTH	As IIa

VI. PITUITARY DISEASES

A. Adenomas

Usually involve anterior lobe, plasma prolactin level usually elevated.

1. Functioning

    a. Growth hormone producing (acromegaly) enlargement of hands, jaw, feet, soft tissue; hyperhidrosis, arthritis, hypertrichosis, diabetes, hypertension, cardiac disease.

    b. ACTH producing (Cushing's disease not syndrome).

        Diagnose with high dose dexamethasone suppression test (8 mg), MRI.

        Treat with transsphenoidal microsurgery.

2. Nonfunctioning - present with space-occupying lesion or hypopituitarism.

    a. Symptoms - headache, tunnel vision due to pressure on optic chiasm.

    b. Signs - papilledema, visual field cuts, erosion of floor of sella; hypogonadism.

3. Surgical treatment - preferred. Adenoma may recur; hypopituitarism may occur.

4. Radiation therapy - may not stop tumor growth indefinitely.

5. Replacement therapy:

    a. Hydrocortisone

    b. Thyroid

    c. Mineralocorticoid therapy usually not required as aldosterone secretion is independent of ACTH.

    d. Sex steroid

B. Neurohypophysis

1. Diabetes insipidus

   a. sarcoidosis

   b. the histiocytoses (eosinophilic granuloma)

   c. post op neurosurgery

   d. neoplasms

   e. patients fail to concentrate urine, get hypernatremic which leads to symptoms of thirst, polydipsia, polyuria.

   f. replace with vasopressin

C. Craniopharyngioma

1. Congenital - Rathke's pouch squamous cell tumors. Suprasellar, may extend into sella; cystic.

2. Calcification - on x-ray

3. Diagnosis - by CT scan. Increased intracranial pressure presents with visual loss secondary to optic papilledema or atrophy. Endocrinopathies as hypogonadism, diabetes insipidus, hypothalamic syndromes as obesity, anorexia.

4. Treatment - surgical but may be incomplete.

D. Hypopituitarism

Multiple endocrine deficiencies.

1. Symptoms - fatigue, weight loss, weakness (asthenia), headache, visual loss, loss of libido, cold intolerance.

2. Signs - absence of axillary and pubic hair, fine facial wrinkling, pallor.

3. Etiologies - neoplasm, vascular (infarction), infection (TB), infiltration (sarcoid).

4. Treatment - try to treat the etiology. Replace hormones. Remember to increase steroid coverage for stress.

VII. ADRENAL GLAND

A. Cushing's Syndrome

Adrenal adenoma (note similarities to and differences from Addison's)

1. Symptoms - weakness, weight gain; hyperglycemic symptoms of polyuria, polydipsia

2. Signs - moon facies, buffalo hump, truncal obesity, hypertension, hypokalemia, hyperglycemia, osteoporosis, no eosinophils

3. Cushing's Syndrome: Iatrogenic. Common in steroid treated patients with COPD, rheumatic diseases. Skin purpura and tendency to easy injury are common. Weight gain and purple striae are cosmetic concerns. Hypertension and hyperglycemia need treatment.

4. Cushing's Syndrome: Ectopic. Due to small cell lung cancer most often. Patients present with weakness and hypokalemia; the metabolic problems are more striking than the physical findings (they may not any have body fat to redistribute to a buffalo hump!)

B. Adrenogen Producing Conditions

1. Virilization - seen with adrenal carcinomas, due to elevated 17-ketosteroids; congenital adrenal hyperplasia usually secondary to impaired C-21 hydroxylation.

2. Adrenal carcinoma - differentiated from adenoma by size; elevated urinary 17-hydroxysteroids and 17-ketosteroids

C. Addison's Disease

1. Symptoms - weakness, weight loss, orthostatic dizziness, anorexia, nausea, vomiting.

2. Signs - hyperpigmentation of skin (melanin) and gums, commonly have vitiligo, skinny vertical heart, dehydration, hypercalcemia, mild renal insufficiency, hypoglycemia, hyperkalemia, eosinophilia, hyperacusis, calcium deposited in pinna.

3. Etiologies - autoimmune most common; metastatic cancer to adrenal is frequent but <u>rarely</u> causes insufficiency or needs treatment.

4. Diagnosis - serum cortisol decreased; serum ACTH increased, cortrosyn stimulation test shows intact pituitary - adrenal axis by a doubling of baseline cortisol.

5. Distinguishing from pituitary causes - hyperpigmentation results from excess ACTH/MSH produced in an attempt to stimulate adrenal. In adrenal failure secondary to pituitary disease, there is no ACTH/MSH and no hyperpigmentation.

6. Treatment - treat any precipitating event. Treat crisis with saline, glucose, and IV hydrocortisone. Chronic therapy will require hydrocortisone and mineralocorticoid. Treatment will also include prophylactic increase in dose of steroids for any major stress, illness, or surgery.

VIII. SEX HORMONES/GLANDS

A. Female

1. Dysgerminomas (rare)

2. Ovarian cancer - no screening test. Presents late, often with ascites. Surgically debulk, use chemotherapy.

3. Disorders related to menopause.

   a. Hot flashes related to autonomic/vascular instability.

   b. Osteoporosis - prevent with estrogens if not contraindicated due to estrogen sensitive cancer.

   c. Vulvar atrophy.

   d. Acceleration of coronary disease - prevent with estrogen.

B. Male

    1. Testicular atrophy

        a. anabolic steroids

        b. post infections

        c. alcohol

    2. Impotence - often psychogenic, may be secondary to diabetes, peripheral vascular disease, testicular failure, treatments for prostate cancer (orchiectomy, estrogen therapy, leuprolide).

IX. QUESTIONS

1. The causes of increased gap metabolic acidosis include (multiple true-false)

    a. methanol ingestion
    b. ethylene glycol ingestion
    c. diabetic ketoacidosis
    d. lactic acidosis
    e. paraldehyde

2. The most common cause of syndrome of inappropriate ADH from a tumor source is

    a. small-cell carcinoma of the lung
    b. renal carcinoma
    c. colon cancer
    d. thyroid carcinoma
    e. breast cancer

3. Common associations with hypothyroidism include (multiple true-false)

    a. hyperlipidemia
    b. increased CPK levels
    c. lethargy
    d. hypermenorrhea
    e. velvet skin
    f. diarrhea

4. Primary hyperparathyroidism classically has which of the following lab abnormalities?

   a. hypercalcemia and hypophosphatemia
   b. hypercalcemia and hyperphosphatemia
   c. hypocalcemia and hyperphosphatemia
   d. hypocalcemia and hypophosphatemia

5. Which endocrine disease would you most suspect in a patient with hypertension, palpitations, arrhythmias, headaches, pallor, flushing, sweating, and anxiety?

   a. pheochromocytoma
   b. Conn's adrenal adenoma
   c. Cushing's syndrome
   d. Addison's disease

6. The leading precipitant of diabetic ketoacidosis is

   a. infection
   b. peptic ulcer disease
   c. cholelithiasis
   d. silent myocardial infarction

7. Initial treatment of the comatose patient should include

   a. maintaining patent airway
   b. bolus of concentrated glucose solution (D50)
   c. Naloxone therapy
   d. all of the above

X. ANSWERS

1. a-True; b-True; c-True; d-True; e-True

2. a

3. a-True; b-True; c-True; d-True; e-False; f-False

4. a

5. a

6. a

7. d

CHAPTER 12:   DRUGS AND THEIR INTERACTIONS

I.   QUESTIONS

1. When starting a hypertensive diabetic on an ACE inhibitor with atherosclerosis you would monitor: (multiple true-false)

    a. Serum K+ (likely to go up)
    b. Serum K+ (likely to go down)
    c. Serum creatinine which may go up, especially if a component of renal artery stenosis exists
    d. Serum creatinine which may go down if pre-existing heart failure improves
    e. Repeated BP measurements

2. A 65 year old black male received dexamethasone as an IV premedication for chemotherapy, followed by oral tablets for 3 days. He experienced late onset nausea and vomiting at 5 days and presented in stupor at 7 days. He was hypo- tensive with minimal urine output. He was afebrile and had a normal white blood cell count. CO2 20, glucose 985, creat 2.6.

    His overall picture is BEST explained by:

    a. Chemotherapy induced sepsis
    b. Chemotherapy induced renal failure
    c. Cerebral edema from brain metastases
    d. Dexamethasone induced diabetic ketoacidosis
    e. Dexamethasone induced diabetic hyperosmolar coma

3. The following are side effects of Prednisone: (multiple true-false)

a. Leukocytosis
b. Eosinophilia
c. Osteopenia
d. Dyspepsia
e. Euphoria
f. Cataracts
g. Hyperglycemia
h. Fat redistribution
i. Hypokalemia
j. Hypercalcemia
k. Anorexia

4. Constipation is a side effect of which of the following? (multiple true-false)

a. Cholestyramine
b. Lomotil
c. Calcium
d. Digitalis
e. Verapamil
f. Quinidine
g. Morphine
h. Sulcralfate
i. Amitriptyline

5. A 55-year-old white male presents with gynecomastia.

You should consider: (multiple true-false)

a. Cimetidine use
b. Ketoconazole use
c. Digoxin use
d. Aldactone use
e. Estrogen use
f. Lung cancer
g. Testicular atrophy
h. Testicular tumor
i. Heart failure
j. Liver disease
k. Kidney disease

6. A patient is referred to you for iron deficiency with no obvious bleeding source on GI x-rays. You note in his old records prior surgery on stomach (gastrectomy) and heart (aortic valve replacement).

The following are in his differential diagnosis: (multiple true-false)

a. Colon polyps not seen on barium enema
b. Iron deficiency from prior gastrectomy
c. Bleeding hemorrhoids
d. Hemochromatosis
e. Blood donor
f. Hereditary hemorrhagic telangiectasia
g. Angiodysplasia
h. Paroxysmal nocturnal hemoglobinuria

7. Neutropenia is a complication of all but one of the following EXCEPT:

   a. Propylthiouracil
   b. Ticlid
   c. Ganciclovir
   d. Azidothymidine
   e. Bleomycin
   f. Captopril
   g. Clozapine

8. Phenytoin can cause all of the following EXCEPT:

   a. Seizures
   b. Lymphadenopathy
   c. Nystagmus
   d. Folate deficiency
   e. Gingival hyperplasia
   f. Stevens-Johnson syndrome
   g. Congestive heart failure

9. What drug can cause the orange man syndrome? (one BEST answer)

   a. Doxorubicin
   b. Rifampin
   c. Vitamin C
   d. Azo Gantrisin
   e. Amphotericin B

10. What drug can cause the gray baby syndrome? (one BEST answer)

   a. Cephalexin
   b. Metronidazole
   c. Chloramphenicol
   d. Penicillin G
   e. Tetracycline

11. All of the following cause very dark urine EXCEPT:

   a. Melaninuria from widespread melanoma
   b. Alkaptonuria
   c. Intermittent porphyria
   d. Rhabdomyolysis
   e. Porphyria cutanea tarda
   f. Hepatorenal syndrome

12. Which of the following causes hemolysis in G-6-P-D deficient individuals? (multiple true-false)

   a. Penicillin
   b. Fava beans
   c. Trimethoprim-sulfa
   d. Dapsone
   e. Methyldopa

13. What causes "silver stools"? (one BEST answer)

   a. Silver nitrate nose drops
   b. Inborn error of metabolism with accumulation of silver in the liver
   c. Acholic stools from common duct obstruction due to ampullary carcinoma with GI bleeding
   d. Living in a silver mining region

14. What causes the skin to be green? (one BEST answer)

   a. Excess ingestion of chlorophyll
   b. Post lymphangiogram lymphangitic spread of marker dye
   c. Post radiation spread of marker tattoo
   d. Use of IVP dye in a jaundiced patient

15. What causes headache, blurred vision, and papilledema (pseudotumor cerebri)? (multiple true-false)

   a. Tetracycline
   b. Vitamin A to excess
   c. Vitamin E to excess
   d. Polar bear liver ingestion by Eskimos
   e. Idiopathic in young women

16. Which of the following causes pigment gallstones? (multiple true-false)

   a. Sickle cell anemia
   b. Thalassemia major
   c. Hereditary spherocytosis
   d. Hereditary elliptocytosis
   e. Porphyria cutanea tarda

17. Which of the following causes blue sclerae? (one BEST answer)

    a. Osteosarcoma
    b. Osteonecrosis
    c. Methylene blue "rescue" after cyanide toxicity
    d. Osteogenesis imperfecta
    e. Osteoid osteoma

18. Which of the following causes orange skin and white sclerae? (one BEST answer)

    a. Excess beets
    b. Excess carrots
    c. Excess broccoli
    d. Excess animal fat

19. Which of the following intravenous infusions can lead to cyanide toxicity? (one BEST answer)

    a. Isoproterenol
    b. Dobutamine
    c. Dopamine
    d. Nitroprusside
    e. Lidocaine

20. Urinary retention can be seen with which of the following? (multiple true-false)

    a. Amitriptyline
    b. Morphine
    c. Flexeril
    d. Prazosin
    e. Atropine

21. Which of the following causes SIADH? (multiple true-false)

    a. Small cell carcinoma
    b. Vincristine
    c. Cyclophosphamide
    d. Morphine
    e. Pain
    f. Lithium
    g. Chlorpropamide

22. The following can cause deafness: (multiple true-false)

   a. Erythromycin
   b. Gentamicin
   c. Cephalexin
   d. Furosemide
   e. Cisplatinol
   f. Hydrochlorothiazide

23. The following can cause visual loss: (multiple true-false)

   a. Hydroxychloroquine
   b. Chloroquine
   c. Isoniazid
   d. Ethambutol
   e. Amiodarone

24. Hypothyroidism can be caused by: (multiple true-false)

   a. Not enough iodine
   b. Lithium
   c. Radioactive iodine
   d. Amiodarone
   e. Propylthiouracil
   f. Digoxin

25. A presumptive cause is found in what percentage of seizure work-ups?

   a. 90 percent
   b. 75 percent
   c. 50 percent
   d. 20-25 percent

26. Common side-effects of phenytoin (Dilantin) treatment are

   a. nystagmus
   b. gingival hyperplasia
   c. osteomalacia
   d. peripheral neuropathy
   e. all of the above

27. Which of the following alcohol withdrawal syndromes are most ominous?

    a. tremulousness
    b. hallucinosis
    c. seizures
    d. delirium tremens
    e. all of the above

28. Instituting acetylcysteine (Mucomyst) should be considered in acute overdose of acetaminophen in which situation?

    a. when one gram ingestion is encountered
    b. two grams of ingestion
    c. four grams of ingestion
    d. ten grams or greater

II. ANSWERS

1. a-True; b-False; c-True; d-True; e-True

2. e

3. a-True; b-False; c-True; d-True; e-True; f-True; g-True; h-True; i-True; j-False; k-False

4. a-True; b-True; c-True; d-False; e-True; f-False; g-True; h-True; i-True

5. a-True; b-True; c-True; d-True; e-True; f-True; g-True; h-True; i-False; j-True; k-False

6. a-True; b-True; c-True; d-False; e-True; f-True; g-True; h-True

7. e

8. g

9. b

10. c

11. e

12. a-False; b-True; c-True; d-True

13. c

14. b

15. a-True; b-True; c-True; d-True; e-True

16. a-True; b-True; c-True; d-True; e-False

17. d

18. b

19. d

20. a-True; b-True; c-True; d-False; e-True

21. a-True; b-True; c-True; d-True; e-True; f-False; g-True

22. a-True; b-True; c-False; d-True; e-True; f-False

23. a-True; b-True; c-False; d-True; e-True

24. a-True; b-True; c-True; d-True; e-True; f-False

25. d

26. e

27. d

28. d